Weight Watchers Instant Pot Cookbook

Weight Watchers Program To Rapid Weight Loss And Better Your Life With 120 Easy And Delicious Smart Points Recipes For Your Instant Pot Pressure Cooker Cooking

David Lee

Table of Contents

Introduction

Hi readers, this is David Lee. At first, thank you and congratulate you for choosing this book "*Weight Watchers Instant Pot Cookbook- Weight Watchers Program To Rapid Weight Loss And Better Your Life With 120 Easy And Delicious Smart Points Recipes For Your Instant Pot Pressure Cooker Cooking*". Wish this book will deliver good information you are looking for!

We all want to lose weight from time to time, but do you ever find that it just goes right back on as soon as you try and go back to normal? That is because the changes you made were not designed for long term use. When we go on a diet normally, our weight crashes down, then we stop dieting, start eating the way we used to, and the weight piles back on again.

The problem is that most diets are either unhealthy or unfair to follow forever. You would get very ill if you followed the cabbage soup diet for too long, and you would be very sad if you couldn't eat cake once in a while. What is more, preparing meals can get very tiresome, and counting calories can be a complete and utter nightmare.

In this book we have combined the Instant Pot and Weight Watchers program in order to provide you a perfect solution for losing weight and improving your lifestyle.

By following Weight Watchers program, you're not just limited to a diet. It comes complete with an exercise plan, a support package, and the option to attend regular meet ups and use online forums, for the community element that so many people love. The Weight Watchers plan means you can control your calories easily, without giving up the foods you truly love. You can even lose weight, increase weight or keep the weight by following it. It is up to you!

An Instant Pot is a wonderful device when it comes to cooking. It allows you to cook complex meals quickly, easily, safely, and economically. It is a multicooker that allows you to pressure cook, slow cook, make yoghurt, boil eggs, steam vegetables, and even steam breads and cakes, all at the press of a button! By using an Instant Pot, you will not only have your favorite delicious foods, but also it will save you too much time and money! Your Instant Pot means you can cook delicious, healthy meals at home, even if you don't have a lot of time or many cooking skills.

Inside this book, you will know all the essential knowledge of weight watchers program and instant pot cooking. By following this book, you will be professional about instant pot using and can control your weight easily! Meantime you will have 120 simple and delicious instant pot recipes, which all have the smart points. You will find: **_Chicken, Beef, Pork, Lamb, Seafood, Vegan & Vegetarian, Soups and Desserts recipes._** With so many flavored smart points recipes, you will plan your eating amount very easy, so control your weight very effectively!

By reading this book, you have a perfect plan for anyone who wants to lose weight, gain weight, or maintain their weight, no matter what your cooking skills, physical abilities, time, or tastes in food.

Best wishes for you!

Chapter 1: Weight Watchers

Overview of the Weight Watchers Diet

When it comes to losing a few pounds, there is no diet plan more established or respected than Weight Watchers. As of the start of 2018, Weight Watchers is 53 years old, and other than a few minor updates to reflect the progress of calorie science, it has barely changed since its creation!

The original idea behind Weight Watchers was to offer a diet plan that made it simple to choose healthy foods, by transforming protein, fat, carbohydrate, and fibre balances into easy to understand smart points. Using the plan a person could enjoy a set amount of point to lose weight, gain weight, or maintain weight, making it one of the very first lifestyle change programs! Not only that, but it was one of the very first diets you could truly personalize, allowing you to use the system, but according to your own body and needs. No more strict meal plans, no more unsustainable crash diets, no more feeling like rubbish, and no more excluding people for being on a special diet for ethical, religious, or health reasons.

And you're not just limited to a diet. It comes complete with an exercise plan, a support package, and the option to attend regular meet ups and use online forums, for the community element that so many people love. Finally, if you have a hard time planning meals and cooking, you can even eat ready meals and pre-prepared foods on this diet! Not only have Weight Watchers teams and followers calculated the points for many brands, but they even have their own range of pre-calculated, measured foods, so anyone can do it.

All Kinds of Weight Watchers Plans

Weight Watchers offers a wide range of plans depending on your financial and support needs. For people who do not have money to spend, there are many free resources available online. They may not offer you the complete experience, but a basic points chart should help you monitor your diet more easily than you would if you had to calorie count or follow a more rigid plan.

If you need minimal support and are happy to spend a little money, **OnlinePlus** is the plan you need. For only a few dollars a week you can follow the Weight Watchers program 100% online. They have a simple app and website where you can access thousands of recipes, set your daily goals, record your progress, look up points, and chat with the community.

If you need full support, then your best option is **Personal Coaching**. Here you will get all the benefits of an OnlinePlus account, with the added benefit of having a professional coach design you a perfect diet and exercise plan, and give you unlimited phone call and message support, to ensure you are meeting your goals, are comfortable, and are informed.

For the best of both worlds, you might want to consider **Meetings + OnlinePlus**. You will still get all the benefits of an OnlinePlus account, but you will also enjoy in-person meetings once a week, lead by a Weight Watchers expert who has used the plan to successfully lose weight.

In 2017 Weight Watchers introduced their **WWFreestyle**, a more flexible plan. This plan is focused on reducing food cravings and includes over 200 foods that are considered zero points, allowing you to be much more relaxed with your diet and still lose weight.

What are Smart Points?

Smart Points are Weight Watchers' own patented way of monitoring the nutritional value of your foods. They adhere to the simple recipe for weight loss or maintenance of calories in vs calories out. So the end goal is to eat as many calories as you need to achieve your goal weight. Rather than starving yourself or accidentally overeating then undereating, the idea is to stick to a set number of points every day, allowing you to gain, lose, or maintain weight safely.

Because calories aren't the only thing that matters, Weight Watchers adds or removes points from food based on its nutritional value. If a food is higher in fibre, higher in micronutrients, lower in sugars, or lower in fat, it will have points deducted. If a food is empty calories, fatty, sugary, or otherwise processed, then it will have points added. The end result is a system that not only helps you track your calories quickly and easily, but encourages you to eat healthy calories!

What is more, Weight Watchers allows 35 flexible points every week. This allows you to have the odd treat, or have a bad day, without feeling too guilty about it. It is recommended that you save these 35 points unless you are really tempted, rather than go all out on the first day, though!

With the new development of WWFreestyle, there are now over 200 foods that are zero points, allowing you to eat them to your heart's content. These foods have been chosen for being low in calories, full of nutrition, and very satisfying, meaning that if you had a bad day or a bad week you can still enjoy a filling meal without ruining your plan.

Advantages and Disadvantages of Smart Points

There are some clear advantages and disadvantages to using a system like Smart Points. The most obvious advantages are:
1. You do not need to count calories. Because your points system substitutes the calorie system, you don't need to count calories any more. And because points are simpler than calories, you no longer need to count in hundreds and thousands.
2. You do not need to worry about your macros. Because your points system counts calories and adjusts for macros, and the diet plans try and make sure you eat a healthy, balanced diet, you no longer need to worry about how much fat, protein, or carbohydrate you are getting.
3. You can follow the same plan for maintenance. When you are done losing weight, you don't have to go back to the old diet that made you fat in the first place. You just increase your points allowance until you stabilize. Likewise if you needed to gain weight.
4. You can follow the plan no matter what your dietary requirements. Vegan, vegetarian, Halal, Kosher, gluten free, dairy free, Paleo, diabetic... whatever diet you are following for whatever reason, the points system allows you to stick to it whilst losing weight.
5. You will eat healthier. Because the points system adds points for unhealthy food and subtracts them from healthy food, you will be

encouraged to eat healthier to make your points go further.

The most obvious disadvantages to the plan are:
1. You need to be following Weight Watchers to get the most up to date plan. Although there are many online resources, you will need to be a member to access the latest plans and points calculators.
2. You may need personal support to work out your ideal plan. If your goals or your health needs are very specific, then you may need the Personal Coaching plan to help you create a plan that will work for you.
3. You still need to count and measure. Unlike with some diets that focus on food types or pre-prepared meals, you still need to count points and weigh foods on Weight Watchers. That is, unless you stick entirely to Weight Watchers foods and ready meals.

That said, the advantages outweigh the disadvantages by quite a bit!

Quick Reference Smart Points Value List

It can be difficult to make calculations all the time. Even if you are following the Weight Watchers points system, sometimes you might be in a rush, or trying to make a traditional or family meal, and not have the time or energy to calculate all the points. For times like these, here are two reliable cheat sheets.

COMMON FOODS LIST		
FOOD	**AMOUNT**	**POINTS**
Bread	1 slice	2
Potato	1 cup	4
Rice	1 cup	5
Apple	1	0
Banana	1	0
Mango	1	0
Orange	1	0
Pear	1	0

Peach	1	0
Watermelon	1 cup	0
Milk, 1%	1 cup	3
Milk, 2%	1 cup	4
Milk, whole	1 cup	5
Yoghurt	1 cup	6
Butter	1 tsp	3
Egg	1	0
Lettuce	1 cup	0
Tomato	1 cup	0
Cucumber	1 cup	0
Beef	2oz	2
Chicken	2oz	3
Fish	6oz	7
Pork	2oz	6
Shrimp	2oz	1
Caesar salad	3 cups	9
Cheeseburger	1 medium	12
Chocolate	1oz	4
Hamburger	1 medium	9
Pizza	1 5oz slice	11
Sandwich	1	15
Apple juice	1 cup	3
Beer	1 can	5

Cola	1 cup	5
Diet Cola	1 cup	0
Orange juice	1 cup	4

CALORIES LIST

CALORIES	POINTS
0-20	0
20-35	1
36-89	2
90-119	3
120-159	4
160-199	5
200-225	6
226-259	7
260-299	8
300-329	9
330-365	10
366-399	11
400-439	12
440-469	13
470-505	14
506-540	15
541-579	16
580-610	17
611-645	18
646-679	19
680-715	20
716-749	21
750-789	22

790-820	23
821-855	24
856-889	25
890-925	26
926-959	27
960-999	28
1000-1029	29
1030-1100	30

These charts are just rough estimates for when you are in a rush and are not the official Weight Watchers listings!

How to Calculate Smart Points

If you haven't got the app handy but you want a more accurate points calculation on the go, there are ways of doing this too! Again, this chart is not absolutely precise. However it might help you if you are in a pinch.

If more than 3g of fibre, remove a point. If less than 1g of fibre, add a point.

FAT → CAL	0g	2g	4g	8g	10g	12g	14g	16g	18g	20g	22g
25	0	0	0	1	1	1	1	1	1	2	2
50	1	1	1	1	1	1	2	2	2	2	2
75	1	1	1	2	2	2	2	2	2	3	3
100	2	2	2	2	2	2	3	3	3	3	3
125	2	2	2	3	3	3	3	3	3	4	4
150	3	3	3	3	3	3	4	4	4	4	4
175	3	3	3	4	4	4	4	4	4	5	5
200	4	4	4	4	4	4	5	5	5	5	5

225	4	4	4	5	5	5	5	5	5	6	6
250	5	5	5	5	5	5	6	6	6	6	6
275	5	5	5	6	6	6	6	6	6	7	7
300	6	6	6	6	6	6	7	7	7	7	7
325	6	6	6	7	7	7	7	7	7	8	8
350	7	7	7	7	7	7	8	8	8	8	8
375	7	7	7	8	8	8	8	8	8	9	9
400	8	8	8	8	8	8	9	9	9	9	9
425	8	8	8	9	9	9	9	9	9	10	10
450	9	9	9	9	9	9	10	10	10	10	10
475	9	9	9	10	10	10	10	10	10	11	11
500	10	10	10	10	10	10	11	11	11	11	11

Is Weight Watchers really effective for weight loss?

It is natural to be sceptical of any diet plan, especially one that will cost you money! Fortunately, not only has Weight Watchers been around for over half a century, but it has plenty of anecdotal and *statistical* evidence that it works. Yes, they have done studies, following thousands of people!

The conclusion of all this research is that the average person loses around 4lbs. If that doesn't seem like much, remember that most people don't have a lot to lose! A fifth of people doing Weight Watchers were found to have lost 5% of their body weight. That means that Weight Watchers members are 8 times more likely to lose 5-10% of their body weight than people trying to lose weight on their own.

The keys? A simple system and support! When you don't need to overthink things, and you have a community of people who are going through the same process with you, you will find it much easier to stick to a plan, and therefore to lose weight.

The science behind Weight Watchers

So how exactly do you lose weight on Weight Watchers? The science is ridiculously simple: calories in must be fewer than calories out. A calorie is a unit of energy, and there are four in each gram of protein or carbohydrate, nine in each gram of fat, and seven in each gram of alcohol. If you eat more calories than you use in a day, your body might lose some of it in your urine or feces, but a lot of it will be stored as fat. If you eat the same amount, you will maintain your weight. If you eat less, you will lose weight!

Even if you suffer a metabolic problem, the solution is still the same. For example, people with Prader-Willi syndrome only burn 700-1300 calories a day. So how do they lose weight? They have to eat 600 calories a day. Naturally, this is easier said than done. You have to control your appetite and count your calories, or your points, closely. But if you achieve the deficit, you will lose weight.

Almost any diet, if it achieves a calorie deficit, can make you lose weight. The trick is sticking to it! Many people find diets hard to stick to because they have cravings, because certain foods are eliminated, because the diet has too much junk food, or because the diet has too few calories. If you go on a diet like the cabbage soup diet, you are bound to feel ill and tired and hungry all day. Which means you will eventually quit!

What Weight Watchers does is it makes following your diet really easy. Firstly, by removing the bothersome figures of calories. Calories are counted in the hundreds and thousands for many foods and most meals. And humans just can't think that high! Can you imagine four hundred oranges? Or do you just picture a pile of oranges? Now imagine 8-9 oranges. Easy, right? That is what Weight Watchers does to calories: it breaks them down into simple figures you can follow easily.

Next, you are encouraged to eat healthy, filling foods. No more living off salads. And no more eating junk food "if it fits your macros"! Weight Watchers allows you to eat almost any food you like, as long as you stick within your points. But there is a catch: you use fewer points on healthy food and more points on unhealthy food. So for the same points, you could eat 100 calories of meat, 600 calories of fruit, or 20 calories of chocolate. This encourages you to fill your belly with nutrients, protein, and fibre.

Finally, you are given a little freedom. You have a 35 point weekly allowance for if you want to eat something truly indulgent. You could go out for dinner and have almost anything you want, have a small dessert every day, or eat a huge festive meal for those points! Not only that, but if you exercise more you can add more points to your day, and there are zero point foods that you can eat endlessly if you really need to fill up.

And when you have lost the weight? All you have to do is increase your point allowance to maintain your weight. You could stay on Weight Watchers for the rest of your life, if you wanted!

What should you eat?

Part of the beauty of Weight Watchers is that really, you can eat whatever you want to. As long as it stays within your points limits, you can eat chocolate cake, or you can eat salad. The points system is designed to persuade you to eat more healthy foods, but it can't *force* you to eat them. If you are a really picky eater, have special dietary requirements, or love certain foods, you can basically follow your normal diet, just adjusting the amount you eat to fit into the points system.

Many people love indulging with zero points foods. This is because the lack of points provides you with a guilt-free pleasure, and because zero points foods are carefully chosen to be nutritious and filling, you will feel satisfied and great physically after eating them too! If you have a hard time controlling your snacking, keeping a supply of zero points snacks could really help you.

That said, it is advisable to try and stick to your points when you can, rather than repeatedly eating under your allowance. Some people stick under their allowance to speed up weight loss, but there is always the risk that you will eat too little and make yourself so hungry you quit the diet. So try and get to around your points limit, if not at or above it.

If you have a hard time counting points, you might find it easier to make use of Weight Watchers branded foods. They come with the points already calculated and printed on the package, so you just pick them up and eat them. Another great method, however, is to create a list of "go to" recipes from this book, so you always know what you are eating, how to make it, and what points it has!

What foods you should avoid

Again, there is no real need to avoid any foods! You can eat whatever you want, and no food is off limits for being "too naughty", "too calorific", or "too fatty and sugary". This lack of restrictions is precisely what makes Weight Watchers so enjoyable for many dieters: You don't need to wait for a "cheat day" to have a slice of cake, a fried breakfast, or a meal out. You can just have it and add the points to your daily record.

That said, not all foods are created equal. You may want to avoid particularly high points foods. This is because they are almost always high in calories, high in fat, high on the glycemic index, high in sugar, low in fibre, low in protein, and generally not at all filling. If you eat all your points in chocolate, for example, you might have only had 5-7oz of chocolate. Which is not enough to keep you full all day!

For the same reason, avoid points drinks. Just like drinking your calories, drinking your points is an easy way to waste them. You will not feel full, you will not feel good, and you will be able to eat less to fill yourself up later on. Instead, choose zero points drinks and save your points for nutritious food.

Likewise, if you have any foods you can't control yourself around, especially if they are zero points foods, you may want to skip them entirely. An apple or an egg might be zero points, but they are still fifty and a hundred calories. The idea is that they are super filling so you will not want or need to binge on them. But if you can eat twenty apples or ten eggs in one day, that is a thousand calories just on snacks! If you have trouble binging, you might want to avoid all zero points foods completely, or assign them points using the calorie charts above.

Chapter 2: Instant Pot

Why Instant Pot?

An Instant Pot is a wonderful device when it comes to cooking. It allows you to cook complex meals quickly, easily, safely, and economically. It is a multicooker that allows you to pressure cook, slow cook, make yoghurt, boil eggs, steam vegetables, and even steam breads and cakes, all at the press of a button!

Quick
It is a much faster way of cooking because it can cook everything in one go, in one pot. If you use the pressure cooking mode it uses high pressure steam and high temperatures to cook your food to perfection in a tenth of the time of conventional cooking methods. If you use the slow cooking mode you can just empty your food into the Instant Pot, seal it, and leave it to cook over several hours. What is more, because you use fewer pots and pans, you save time on clean up as well!

Easy
It is so simple to use! Just put the ingredients in your Instant Pot, seal it, select the right mode, and it will cook your food for you. It does not involve many different steps, it does not take up much space on your counter, and it even has a timer and a warming function so that you do not need to worry about overcooking your food, or food getting cold as you wait for people to arrive for dinner.

Safe
Unlike conventional cooking methods, the Instant Pot keeps almost all the heat and oil away from you. Because it is sturdy on the counter, there is little to no risk of tipping it. And because it has a pressure gauge and automatic pressure release settings, you can handle it safely, knowing that the Instant Pot will not allow you to come in contact with hot steam and boiling liquids. Its design also makes it perfect for people with mobility issues, people with cognitive problems, and children to use, although always supervised.

Economical

Although buying your Instant Pot may seem expensive, in the long run it will save you money. Because you do not need to use other pots, pans, or kitchen equipment most of the time, you can save money on maintaining and replacing these tools. And because you are cooking your own meals in minutes, you can save money on ready meals and fast food.

The buttons and features

So how does this amazing machine work? It may seem a little intimidating at first glance, but rest assured it is not all that complicated! All of its buttons come labelled with their functions, and after a short while you will be using it as easily as you use your phone.

Soup: A high pressure cook for 30 min, that will draw the moisture out of vegetable to make a delicious soup or stock.

Meat/Stew: A high pressure cook for 35 min, which properly breaks down protein, fat, sinew, and fibre.

Bean/Chili: A high pressure cook for 30 min which will soak and cook your legumes.

Poultry: A high pressure 15 minute cook time that will get your poultry to temperature, but not dry out the white meat.

Rice: A low pressure fully automatic program that will cook white or brown rice and other husk-free grains.

Multi-grain: A high pressure 40 minute cook time, great for wild rice and other whole grains.

Porridge: A high pressure 20 minute cook time which will produce great porridge, tapioca, and grain puddings.

Slow Cook: A low pressure setting that allows you to cook your food over a longer period of time, for a delicious complete meal.

Steam: A high pressure 10 minute   cook time, perfect for heating water just high enough to provide steam to cook things in.

Cake: A button for cheesecakes and other moist cakes. It has three different settings depending on the type of cake.

Egg: A button for boiling eggs, with settings from soft to hard boiled.

Sterilize: A high pressure burst of hot steam to sterilize fresh fruit and vegetables and cooking utensils. You can also use it for canning!

You also have plus and minus buttons which you can use to alter the times of these settings and to jiggle the mode, as well as a pressure button to increase or decrease pressure. That said, whilst adjusting the temperature is great, maybe don't play with the pressure too much, as it is often ideal on each setting!

Useful Tips for Using an Instant pot

When using an Instant Pot, try and bear in mind that however safe it is, you are still dealing with very high pressures, very high temperatures, and electricity! If you use your Instant Pot correctly it is the safest thing in the world. But if you use it incorrectly you could still hurt yourself. To make sure you are always safe, follow these steps:

ALWAYS:
- Watch the fill lines. Every Instant Pot model has its own limits, to always make sure to use above the minimum and below the maximum amount of fluid.
- Make sure to count things that liquefy, like sugar or gelatine, as liquids, and measure them by volume.
- Keep your hands away from the steam, as it is very hot!
- Release the pressure according to the recipe and according to your Instant Pot's instructions. Stay safe.
- Check that you have all the right parts. You can't steam without a steamer basket, or cook without your insert!
- Clean your Instant Pot thoroughly. Make sure the insert and steamer basket are clean and nothing is between the Instant Pot unit and the basket. Wipe the main body with a lightly damp or dry cloth when it is cool.

NEVER:
- Put it on the stove top. This is not a conventional pressure cooker, it works electrically. If you put it on the stove you can break it and hurt yourself.
- Cook without your insert. You will break the Instant Pot and risk

electrocution.

- Try a recipe with the wrong pieces. Always use the attachments, baking paper, etc, as instructed, to avoid damaging the Instant Pot.
- Fill it with oil. It is not a deep fat fryer!
- Use the quick release function when not specified. Releasing high pressure too quickly can be very dangerous.
- Leave it unattended. Although you can leave slow cookers cooking at home, your Instant Pot needs someone at home at all times, in case of accidents.
- Force the lid. The pressure is dangerous!

Cooking time for various foods

Different foods have different cooking times in your Instant Pot. Here is a basic guide as to how long to cook some common foods, based on their own instructions.

Rice & Grains	Water Quantity Ratio (grain : water)	Cooking Time
Barley, pearl	1 : 2.5	20 – 22
Congee, thick	1 : 4 – 1 : 5	15 – 20
Congee, thin	1 : 6 – 1 : 7	15 – 20
Couscous	1 : 2	2 – 3
Corn, dried / halved	1 : 3	5 – 6
Oats, quick cooking	1 : 1.5	2 – 3
Oats, steel-cut	2 : 2.5	3 – 5
Porridge, thin	1 : 2	10 – 15
Quinoa, quick cooking	1 : 1.25	1
Rice, Basmati	1 : 1	4
Rice, Brown	1 : 1	22 – 25
Rice, white	1 : 1	4
Rice, wild	1 : 1	20 – 25

Meat	Cooking Time (minutes)
Beef, stew meat	20 / 450 gm / 1 lb
Beef, meat ball	8 – 10 / 450 gm / 1 lb
Beef, dressed	20 / 450 gm / 1 lb
Beef (pot roast, steak, rump, round, chuck, blade or brisket) Small Chunks	15 / 450 gm / 1 lb
Beef (pot roast, steak, rump, round, chuck, blade or brisket) Large Chuncks	20 / 450 gm / 1 lb
Beef, ribs	20 – 25
Beef, shanks	25 – 30
Beef, oxtail	40 – 50
Chicken, breasts (boneless)	6 – 8
Chicken, whole 2-2.5 Kg	8 / 450 gm / 1 lb
Chicken, cut with bones	10 – 15
Chicken, bone stock	40 – 45
Duck, portions with bones	12 – 15
Duck, whole	10 / 450 gm / 1 lb
Ham, slices	9 – 12
Ham, picnic shoulder	8 / 450 gm / 1 lb
Lamb, cubes	10 – 15
Lamb, stew meat	12 – 15
Lamb, leg	15 / 450 gm / 1 lb
Pork, loin roast	20 / 450 gm / 1 lb
Pork, butt roast	15 / 450 gm / 1 lb
Pork, ribs	15 – 20
Turkey, breast (boneless)	7 – 9
Turkey, breast (whole)	20 – 25
Turkey, drumsticks (leg)	15 – 20
Veal, chops	5 – 8
Veal, roast	12 / 450 gm / 1 lb

Seafood & Fish	FRESH Cooking Time (minutes)	FROZEN Cooking Time (minutes)
Crab, whole	2 – 3	4 – 5
Fish, whole	4 – 5	5 – 7
Fish, fillet	2 – 3	3 – 4
Fish, steak	3 – 4	4 – 6
Lobster	3 – 4	4 – 6
Mussels	2 – 3	n/a
Seafood soup or stock	7 – 8	8 – 9
Shrimp or Prawn	1 – 3	2 – 4

Dried Beans, Legumes, and Lentils	DRY Cooking Time (minutes)	SOAKED Cooking Time (minutes)
Adzuki	16 – 20	4 – 6
Black beans	20 – 25	6 – 8
Black-eyed peas	10 – 15	4 – 5
Chickpeas (chickpeas, garbanzo bean, or kabuli)	35 – 40	10 – 15
Cannellini beans	30 – 35	8 – 10
Kidney beans	25 – 30	8 – 10
Lentils, green	10 – 12	n/a
Lentils, red, split	5 – 6	n/a
Lima beans	12 – 14	8 – 10
Pinto beans	25 – 30	8 – 10
Peas	6 – 10	n/a
Soy beans	35 – 45	18 – 20

Vegetables	FRESH Cooking Time (minutes)	FROZEN Cooking Time (minutes)

Artichoke, whole & trimmed	9 – 11	11 – 13
Artichoke, hearts	4 – 5	5 – 6
Asparagus, whole or cut	1 – 2	2 – 3
Beans, green, yellow or wax, whole, trim ends and strings	1 – 2	2 – 3
Beetroot, small / whole	11 – 13	13 – 15
Beetroot, large / whole	20 – 25	25 – 30
Broccoli, florets	1 – 2	2 – 3
Broccoli, stalks	3 – 4	4 – 5
Brussel sprouts, whole	2 – 3	3 – 4
Cabbage, red, purple or green, shredded	2 – 3	3 – 4
Cabbage, red, purple or green, wedges	3 – 4	4 – 5
Carrots, sliced or shredded	2 – 3	3 – 4
Carrots, whole or chunked	6 – 8	7 – 9
Cauliflower florets	2 – 3	3 – 4
Collard Greens	4 – 5	5 – 6
Corn (kernels)	1 – 2	2 – 3
Corn (on the cob)	3 – 5	4 – 6
Eggplant (slices or chunks)	3 – 4	3 – 4
Green beans (whole)	2 – 3	3 – 4
Greens (chopped)	2 – 3	4 – 7
Leeks	2 – 3	3 – 4
Mixed vegetables	3 – 4	4 – 6
Okra	2 – 3	3 – 4
Onions (sliced)	2 – 3	3 – 4
Parsnips (chunks)	3 – 4	4 – 5
Peas (in the pod)	1 – 2	2 – 3
Peas (green)	1 – 2	2 – 3
Potatoes (cubed)	3 – 4	4 – 5
Baby potatoes (whole)	8 – 10	12 – 14
Large potatoes (whole)	12 – 15	15 – 19
Pumpkin (small pieces)	2 – 3	4 – 5

Pumpkin (larges pieces)	8 – 10	10 – 14
Rutabaga (slices)	3 – 4	4 – 5
Rutabaga (chunks)	4 – 6	6 – 8
Spinach	1 – 2	3 – 4
Acorn squash (slices)	6 – 7	8 – 10
Butternut squash (slices)	4 – 6	6 – 8
Sweet Potato (cubes)	3 – 4	4 – 5
Sweet Potato (whole)	12 – 15	17 – 19
Sweet Pepper (slices or chunks)	1 – 3	2 – 4
Tomatoes (quarters)	2 – 3	4 – 5

Fruits	FRESH Cooking Time (minutes)
Apples (slices or pieces)	1 – 2
Apples (whole)	3 – 4
Apicot (whole or halves)	2 – 3
Peaches	2 – 3
Pears (whole)	3 – 4
Pears (slices or halves)	2 – 3

Recipe notes

All these recipes follow the same format, to make them easy to follow if you are on a Weight Watchers diet. You will need to find recipes that suit your own needs, so make sure to check the ingredients before making anything. However in most cases, if the recipe calls for something you do not eat, such as yoghurt, pork, or wheat flour, you can substitute it for an equal amount of an alternative food that has a similar consistency and function.

All the recipes are sorted into categories based on their ingredients and cooking method, so you can find the recipes you need quickly and easily.

Each recipe begins with a title, the number of servings it provides, how long it takes to prepare, and how long it takes to cook. This will allow you to make calculations in advance and make sure it suits your needs.

Next the nutritional values of the recipe are listed. This is the nutrition *per serving*, not for the whole recipe! Included are the calories, Smart Points, fat, protein, and carbohydrate contained in each serving.

Finally there is the list of ingredients you will need for the recipe, followed by the recipe itself. The ingredients follow US measurements and the recipe is plotted out in simple, easy to follow steps.

Measurement Conversion Table

If you have any difficulty with US/Imperial measurements, please refer to this Imperial-Metric-Volume conversion table when cooking:

IMPERIAL	METRIC	CUPS
1oz	28g	8tsp
1lb	453.5	3.5 cups
1fl/oz	29.5ml	6tsp
1 gallon	3.8L	16 cups
0.03 oz	1 gram	0.25tsp
2.2lb	1 kilo	8 cups
0.3fl/oz	1 milliliter	0.2tsp
33.8fl/oz	1 liter	4.2 cups
1 inch	2.54cm	1tbsp
0.4 inch	1 cm	1tsp
0.17fl/oz	5ml	1tsp
0.5fl/oz	15ml	1tbsp
8fl/oz	236.5ml	1 cup

Chapter 3: Delicious Recipes

Chicken

CHICKEN LOAF

Serves: 12
Prep time: 15 min
Cooking time: 30 min

Nutrition:
Calories: 210
Points: 5
F: 10g, P: 23g, C: 4g.

Ingredients:
- 3 lbs diced chicken
- 2 cups herb and onion stuffing crumbs mix
- 1 cup chicken broth
- 4 eggs
- salt and pepper to taste

Recipe:
1. Mix the meat, crumbs, eggs, salt, pepper, in one bowl.
2. Put the Steam rack in your Instant Pot and pour in the broth.
3. Take some aluminium foil and make a loaf before wrapping in the foil.
4. Put your meatloaf on your Steam rack.
5. Cook on Steam for 30 min.
6. Release the pressure quickly and let your meatloaf cool before serving it.

CHICKEN CASSEROLE

Serves: 8
Prep time: 15 min
Cooking time: 3h 30 min

Nutrition:
Calories: 282
Points: 5
F: 10g, P: 21g, C: 26g.

Ingredients:
- 2 cups diced lean chicken breast
- 1 cup chicken stock
- 1 can mushroom soup
- 1 can chopped tomatoes
- 2 diced bell peppers
- 1 diced onion
- 1 tablespoon garlic
- 1 tablespoon chili
- salt and pepper
- 10-15 tortillas
- 8 ounces shredded cheese

Recipe:
1. Mix all ingredients in your Instant Pot other than the tortillas and cheese.
2. Crumble tortillas on top.
3. Cook for 3 and a half hours on Slow Cook.
4. Sprinkle cheese on top and let it melt.

CHICKEN ENCHILADAS

Serves: 8
Prep time: 20 min
Cooking time: 25 min

Nutrition:
Calories: 250
Points: 3
F: 10g, P: 25g, C: 15g.

Ingredients:
- 3 cups diced lean chicken breast
- 3 cans low salt tomato sauce
- ½ cup chile
- 4 chopped red and green peppers
- 1 chopped onion
- 2 cloves chopped garlic
- 1 teaspoon olive oil

Recipe:
1. Heat your Instant Pot up with the oil, onions, and garlic. Cook five minutes to soften.
2. Turn down to low. Add all over ingredients.
3. Cook for 25 minutes on Stew.

CHICKEN PHO

Serves: 6
Prep time: 15 min
Cooking time: 15 min

Nutrition:
Calories: 242
Points: 5
F: 12g, P: 20g, C: 8g.

Ingredients:
- 2lbs chicken, cut into thin strips
- 12oz cubed tofu
- 1 cup chopped mushrooms
- 1 cup chicken stock
- ¼ cup black bean sauce
- ¼ cup oyster sauce

Recipe:
1. Put your Instant Pot on high and add the stock and sauces. Cook for 2 min.
2. Add the chicken and seal.
3. Cook on Stew for 15 min.
4. Release the pressure quickly, add the tofu and mushrooms, seal and cook on Stew for 1 more min.
5. Release the pressure and enjoy.

HOT CHICKEN TACOS

Serves: 4
Prep time: 10 min
Cooking time: 15 min

Nutrition:
Calories: 232
Points: 5
F: 4g, P: 32g, C: 39g.

Ingredients:
- 1lb chopped chicken breast
- 1 ¼ cups gravy stock
- ½ cup minced onions
- ½   cup minced peppers
- 1 tbsp Worcestershire sauce
- 1 tbsp extra virgin olive oil
- 1tbsp smoked paprika
- ¼ tsp cloves, powdered
- 8 soft taco shells

Recipe:
1. Add the oil to your Instant Pot.
2. Soften the onions for 5 min until clear.
3. Sauté the chicken and peppers with the onion.
4. Add the remaining ingredients and mix well.
5. Set to Stew and cook on high for 5 min.
6. Release the pressure quickly and serve in taco shells.

CHICKEN BOLOGNESE SAUCE

Serves: 4
Prep time: 15 min
Cooking time: 5h

Nutrition:
Calories: 350
Points: 8
F: 19g, P: 30g, C: 26g.

Ingredients:
- 1lb minced chicken thighs
- 1 pint tomato sauce
- ½ cup minced onions
- 3 tablespoons olive oil
- 1 tablespoon minced garlic
- 2 teaspoons sugar
- salt and pepper
- noodles or zoodles to serve

Recipe:
1. Mix all ingredients other than 1 tablespoon of oil and the noodles in your Instant Pot.
2. Cook for 5 hours on Slow Cook.
3. Cook the noodles or zoodles.
4. Serve.

CHICKEN WITH OLIVES

Serves: 6
Prep time: 5 min
Cooking time: 40 min

Nutrition:
Calories: 275
Points: 6
F: 13g, P: 29g, C: 7g.

Ingredients:
- 4 lbs boneless, skinless chicken thighs
- 2 cans chopped tomato
- ¼ cup pitted black olives
- ¼ cup pitted green olives
- 3 teaspoons paprika
- 1 teaspoon olive oil
- 1 tablespoon minced garlic
- salt and pepper to taste

Recipe:
1. Warm the oil in your Instant Pot.
2. Put the chicken in the Instant Pot to brown.
3. Mix the remaining ingredients together.
4. Pour the sauce over the chicken.
5. Cook on Stew for 40 minutes.

HOT CHICKEN BURRITOS

Serves: 8
Prep time: 20 min
Cooking time: 25 min

Nutrition:
Calories: 250
Points: 5
F: 10g, P: 25g, C: 14g.

Ingredients:
- 3 jars hot tomato sauce
- 3 cups diced chicken, light and dark meat
- 4 chopped mixed peppers
- 1 chopped onion
- ½ cup chile ancho mince
- 2 cloves chopped garlic
- 1 teaspoon olive oil
- 8 flour tortillas

Recipe:
1. Heat your Instant Pot with the oil, onions, chile, and garlic.
2. Cook five minutes until soft.
3. Turn down to low. Add all other ingredients and mix well.
4. Cook on Stew for 25 minutes.
5. Depressurize naturally and serve in burrito wraps.

CHICKEN CHILI

Serves: 6
Prep time: 25 min
Cooking time: 25 min

Nutrition:
Calories: 340
Points: 7
F: 6g, P: 27g, C: 25g.

Ingredients:
- 1 ½lbs minced chicken breast
- 28oz canned tomatoes, chopped
- 17oz chicken stock
- 16oz white beans, canned
- 1 minced onion
- 1 minced red pepper
- 2tbsp smoked paprika
- 1tbsp cinnamon
- 1tbsp worcestershire sauce
- 1tbsp olive oil

Recipe:
1. Put your Instant Pot on high, add the oil and the onion. Soften 5 minutes.
2. Add the other ingredients and mix well.
3. Seal and cook on Stew for 25 min.
4. Release the pressure slowly.

SHREDDED BBQ CHICKEN

Serves: 8
Prep time: 5 min
Cooking time: 6h

Nutrition:
Calories: 166
Points: 3
F: 3g, P: 17g, C: 15g.

Ingredients:
- 24 ounces diced lean chicken breast
- ¾ cup BBQ sauce
- 2 tablespoons brown sugar
- 2 tablespoons chicken broth
- 1 tablespoon Worcestershire sauce
- salt and pepper to taste

Recipe:
1. Mix the sauce in your Instant Pot.
2. Put the chicken in the slow cooker, pour the sauce on top. Cook for 6 hours on Slow Cook.
3. Shred the chicken in the sauce.

CHICKEN SOUP

Serves: 10
Prep time: 10 min
Cooking time: 30 min

Nutrition:
Calories: 20
Points: 0
F: 1g, P: 1g, C: 2g.

Ingredients:
- 1 chicken carcass
- 3 celery stalks, minced
- 2 carrots, minced
- 1 tomato, minced
- 1 onion, minced
- 1 cup chopped frozen peas
- Italian herbs
- salt

Recipe:
1. Put everything but the frozen peas in your Instant Pot. Cover with water.
2. Seal and cook on Stew for 30 minutes.
3. Depressurize naturally.
4. Strain. Press so the cooked veg gets into the soup. Discard the carcass and used veg.
5. Add the frozen peas and simmer until cooked through.

CHICKEN AND SPROUTS

Serves: 5
Prep time: 10 min
Cooking time: 25 min

Nutrition:
Calories: 135
Points: 2
F: 7g, P: 26g, C: 10g.

Ingredients:
- 2lbs chicken breast
- 20 oz chicken stock
- 2 cups beansprouts
- 4 green bell peppers, cut into thin strips
- 1 red onion, cut into thin strips
- 4 garlic cloves, minced
- 4tbsp oyster sauce

Recipe:
1. Mix all the ingredients in your Instant Pot.
2. Set to Stew and cook for 25 minutes.
3. Release the pressure quickly.

TAMARI AND EDAMAME CHICKEN

Serves: 6
Prep time: 25 min
Cooking time: 16 min

Nutrition:
Calories: 235
Points: 4
F: 4g, P: 33g, C: 32g.

Ingredients:
- 2 cups cubed chicken breasts
- 1 diced onion
- 1 diced carrot
- 3 diced scallions
- 1 cup long grain rice, rinsed
- 2/3 cup edamame
- 2/3 cup tamari sauce
- ¼ cup oyster sauce

Recipe:
1. Put the rice in a suitable container in the Steamer basket of your Instant Pot.
2. Mix the remaining ingredients in the base of the Instant Pot.
3. Insert the steamer basket.
4. Cook on Stew for 16 min.
5. Release the pressure naturally and fluff the rice.

CHICKEN THIGH CARNITAS

Serves: 8
Prep time: 15 min
Cooking time: 8h

Nutrition:
Calories: 180
Points: 3
F: 3g, P: 29g, C: 5g.

Ingredients:
- 2lbs boneless, skinless chicken thighs
- ½ cup orange juice
- ½ cup beer
- juice of one lemon and one lime
- 2 tablespoons smoked paprika
- 1 tablespoon black peppercorns
- 1 tablespoon olive oil

Recipe:
1. Rub the chicken with the seasoning mix.
2. Put in your Instant Pot. Pour beer and juices on top.
3. Cook for 8 hours on Slow Cook.
4. Remove and shred.
5. Add some olive oil to the base of your Instant Pot.
6. Stir fry the chicken in it to add some crispiness.

POMODORO CHICKEN

Serves: 6
Prep time: 5 min
Cooking time: 20 min

Nutrition:
Calories: 80
Points: 1
F: 4g, P: 5g, C: 6.5g.

Ingredients:
- 3lbs chicken thighs, bone-in
- 1lb cherry tomatoes
- 1 cup water
- 1/4 cup red wine
- 2 minced garlic cloves
- 1tbsp Italian herbs
- salt and pepper

Recipe:
1. Mix everything in your Instant Pot.
2. Seal and cook on Stew for 20 minutes.

Beef

SHREDDED BEEF.

Serves: 12
Prep time: 15 min
Cooking time: 60 min

Nutrition:
Calories: 310
Points: 7
F: 22g, P: 35g, C: 11g.

Ingredients:
- 3 lbs diced stewing beef
- 2 cups chopped tomato
- 1 minced onion
- 2tbsp Italian herbs
- 2tbsp cayenne
- 2tbsp olive oil
- 2   bay leaves
- salt and pepper to taste

Recipe:
1. Put your Instant Pot on high and add a tbsp of oil.
2. Season the beef with salt and pepper.
3. When the oil is hot, brown the meat and soften the onion 5 min.
4. Cover in the sauce. Add the bay leaves.
5. Seal and cook on Stew for an hour.
6. Depressurise slowly. Remove bay leaves.
7. Shred the beef.

OSSO BUCCO

Serves: 8
Prep time: 30 min
Cooking time: 8h

Nutrition:
Calories: 186
Points: 4
F: 6g, P: 24g, C: 9g.

Ingredients:
- 3lbs beef shank or ox tail
- 2 cups diced onion
- 1 cup chopped carrot
- 1 cup chopped celery
- 1 tin tomatoes
- 8 chopped garlic cloves
- ¼ ounce mushrooms
- ½ cup red wine
- 1 tablespoon oil
- 1tbsp lemon juice
- salt and pepper

Recipe:
1. Put the Instant Pot on high heat with half a tablespoon of oil and the onions.
2. After five minutes, add the remaining oil and the beef.
3. Stir the beef for 10 minutes.
4. Add the remaining ingredients.
5. Cover with stock or water and set to Slow Cook 8 hours.

BOLOGNESE

Serves: 6
Prep time: 15 min
Cooking time: 40 min

Nutrition:
Calories: 338
Points: 8
F: 19g, P: 24g, C: 13g.

Ingredients:
- 1.5 lbs minced beef
- 1.5 cups chopped tomato
- 1.5 cups chopped onion
- 1 cup red wine
- 1 cup beef bone broth
- ½ cup chopped carrot and celery
- 5 minced garlic cloves
- 2 tablespoons Italian herbs
- a bay leaf
- salt, pepper

Recipe:
1. Put some oil in your Instant Pot.
2. Soften the onion 5 minutes.
3. Add the beef. Brown for 10 minutes.
4. Add the remaining ingredients.
5. Cook on Stew for 40 minutes.

RUSTIC STEW

Serves: 6
Prep time: 10 min
Cooking time: 20 min

Nutrition:
Calories: 340
Points: 7
F: 20g, P: 33g, C: 11g.

Ingredients:
- 3 lbs diced beef rump
- 1 marrow bone
- 1 cup tomato passata
- 1 cup stock or gravy
- 1 cup chopped red onion
- 1 cup chopped spring onion
- 2tbsp canola oil
- 2tbsp oregano
- 2   bay leaves
- salt and pepper to taste

Recipe:
1. Put your Instant Pot on High and warm the oil in it.
2. Add the beef, salt and pepper, and red onion.
3. Soften 5 minutes.
4. Add the remaining ingredients.
5. Seal and cook on Stew for 20 minutes.
6. Release the pressure slowly.
7. Throw away the bay leaves and bone.
8. Stir all well.

ONIONY MEATLOAF

Serves: 8
Prep time: 15 min
Cooking time: 30 min

Nutrition:
Calories: 297
Points: 6
F: 11g, P: 32g, C: 22g.

Ingredients:
- 3 lbs 12% fat beef mince
- 2 cups Panko bread crumbs
- 1 cup beef broth
- ½ cup onions
- 4 eggs
- 4tbsp Italian herbs
- salt and pepper to taste

Recipe:
1. Mix the meat, crumbs, eggs, and onions in one bowl.
2. Put the Steam rack in your Instant Pot and pour in the broth.
3. Take some foil and make a loaf with the mince before wrapping in the foil.
4. Put your meatloaf on your Steam rack.
5. Cook on Steam for 30 min.
6. Release the pressure quickly and let your meatloaf cool before serving it.

STEW PROVENCALE

Serves: 6
Prep time: 30 min
Cooking time: 8h

Nutrition:
Calories: 310
Points: 6
F: 8g, P: 32g, C: 26g.

Ingredients:
- 1.5lbs boneless beef
- 1 cup gravy
- 2 onions
- 2 cups carrots
- 3 cups potato
- 8 garlic cloves, crushed
- 2 tbsp plain flour
- 2tbsp herbes de provence
- salt and pepper

Recipe:
1. Roughly dice the meat and vegetables into cubes.
2. Put all ingredients in your Instant Pot.
3. Cook for 8 hours on Slow Cook.

KETO CHILI

Serves: 8
Prep time: 5 min
Cooking time: 50 min

Nutrition:
Calories: 210
Points: 4
F: 10g, P: 22g, C: 11g.

Ingredients:
- 1.5lbs minced beef
- 2 cans tomatoes
- 2 cups diced onion
- 1 cup diced pepper
- 1 cup veg stock
- ½ cup sour cream
- 2 ounces dark chocolate
- 5 chiles
- 2 teaspoons minced garlic
- salt, pepper, cumin to taste

Recipe:
1. Put the oil and onions in your Instant Pot and soften 5 minutes.
2. Add the remaining ingredients and cook on Stew 50 minutes.

FRENCH ONION BEEF

Serves: 5
Prep time: 5 min
Cooking time: 25 min

Nutrition:
Calories: 200
Points: 5
F: 15g, P: 24g, C: 9g.

Ingredients:
- 2lbs beef steak, cubed
- 20 oz beef stock
- ¼ cup white wine
- 2 sweet onions, minced
- 2 red onions, minced
- 4 spring onions, chopped
- 4 garlic cloves, minced
- 1 tbsp Provence seasoning
- salt and pepper

Recipe:
1. Mix all the ingredients in your Instant Pot.
2. Set to Stew and cook for 25 minutes.
3. Release the pressure quickly.

QUICK CHILI

Serves: 6
Prep time: 20 min
Cooking time: 25 min

Nutrition:
Calories: 230
Points: 5
F: 7g, P: 26g, C: 23g.

Ingredients:
- 1 ½lbs beef, ground
- 28oz tomato passata
- 17oz stock
- 2 minced onions
- 8oz red kidney beans
- 8oz cannelini beans
- 2tbsp canola oil

Recipe:
1. Put your Instant Pot on high and add the oil.
2. When the oil is hot, soften the onions and brown the beef.
3. Add the remaining ingredients and mix well.
4. Seal and cook on Stew for 25 min.

MUSHROOM MEATLOAF

Serves: 6
Prep time: 10 min
Cooking time: 5h

Nutrition:
Calories: 275
Points: 6
F: 15g, P: 30g, C: 5g.

Ingredients:
- 1.5lb 11% fat minced beef
- 1.5 cups diced shiitake mushrooms
- 2 eggs
- 1 cup diced onion
- ¼ cup minced garlic
- 2 tablespoons tomato sauce
- 2 teaspoons mustard
- 1 teaspoon thyme
- salt and pepper

Recipe:
1. Combine beef, mushrooms, onion, eggs, garlic, herbs, and salt and pepper.
2. Form a loaf and place into slow cooker.
3. Mix tomato, mustard, and salt and pepper.
4. Spread the tomato mix over the loaf.
5. Cook on Slow Cook 5 hours.

SLOPPY JOE FILLING

Serves: 6
Prep time: 25 min
Cooking time: 10 min

Nutrition:
Calories: 180
Points: 4
F: 6g, P: 15g, C: 3.5g.

Ingredients:
- 1lb ground beef
- 1 cup gravy
- 1 cup tomato passata
- 1 red onion chopped
- 1 bell pepper chopped
- 3tbsp apple cider vinegar
- 1tbsp worcestershire sauce
- 1tsp olive oil
- salt and pepper

Recipe:
1. Heat the oil in your Instant Pot, add the onions and beef and brown for 5 minutes.
2. Add the remaining ingredients.
3. Cook on Stew 10 minutes.

BEEF AND WILD MUSHROOMS

Serves: 4
Prep time:10 min
Cooking time: 18 min

Nutrition:
Calories: 175
Points: 3
F: 6g, P: 27g, C: 13g.

Ingredients:
- 5lbs super lean beef, cut into small cubes
- 13oz beef stock
- 1 yellow onion, chopped
- 1 red onion, chopped
- 1 red pepper, chopped
- 4oz wild mushrooms, sliced
- 2 garlic cloves, minced

Recipe:
1. Put your Instant Pot on high and add the oil.
2. Soften the onions 5 minutes.
3. Put all the ingredients in.
4. Seal and cook on Stew for 18 min.
5. Release the pressure quickly, serve.

VEAL BOLOGNESE

Serves: 6
Prep time: 10 min
Cooking time: 35 min

Nutrition:
Calories: 308
Points: 7
F: 16g, P: 24g, C: 14.5g.

Ingredients:
- 2lbs ground veal
- 1.5 cups tomato puree
- 1.5 cups chopped onion
- 1 cup white wine
- 1 cup beef broth
- ½ cup chopped carrot
- 6 minced garlic cloves
- 2 teaspoons sugar
- 2 tablespoons Italian herbs
- a bay leaf
- salt, pepper

Recipe:
1. Mix all the ingredients in your Instant Pot.
2. Seal and cook on Stew 35 minutes.

BEEF AND CHORIZO

Serves: 4
Prep time: 15 min
Cooking time: 45 min

Nutrition:
Calories: 320
Points: 10
F: 26g, P: 29g, C: 10g.

Ingredients:
- ½ lb rump diced
- 6oz diced chorizo
- 1 onion minced
- 1 carrot chopped
- 1 celery stalk chopped
- ½ cup red wine
- ½ cup beef broth
- 1tbsp olive oil
- 1tbsp smoked paprika
- herbes du provence
- salt and pepper

Recipe:
1. Heat the oil in your Instant Pot and brown the meats all over.
2. Add the onion and soften 5 minutes.
3. Add the remaining ingredients and mix very well.
4. Seal and cook on Stew 45 minutes.

FRENCH BEEF STEW

Serves: 6
Prep time: 5 min
Cooking time: 15 min

Nutrition:
Calories: 620
Points: 12
F: 35g, P: 50g, C: 5g.

Ingredients:
- 2lbs diced brisket
- 1 cup red wine
- 1 cup beef stock
- 1 cup button mushrooms
- 6 carrots cubed
- 1 onion cubed
- 2tbsp minced garlic
- 1tbsp marmite
- cayenne
- salt and pepper

Recipe:
1. Mix all the ingredients in your Instant Pot.
2. Seal and cook on Stew 15 minutes.
3. Depressurize naturally.

Pork

SWEET KETCHUP MEATLOAF

Serves: 8
Prep time: 15 min
Cooking time: 30 min

Nutrition:
Calories: 320
Points: 7
F: 15g, P: 22g, C: 32g.

Ingredients:
- 3 lbs sausage
- 2 cups sage and onion stuffing
- ½ cup ketchup
- ¼ cup light brown sugar
- 4 eggs
- 2tbsp molasses
- 2tbsp onion powder
- salt

Recipe:
1. Mix the meat, crumbs, eggs in one bowl.
2. Mix the sugar, ketchup, molasses, onion, salt in another bowl.
3. Put the Steam rack in your Instant Pot and pour in the broth.
4. Take some aluminium foil and make a loaf.
5. Pour ketchup sauce over before wrapping in the foil.
6. Put your meatloaf on your Steam rack.
7. Cook on Steam for 30 min.
8. Release the pressure quickly and let your meatloaf cool before serving it.

PULLED PORK AND PEACHES

Serves: 12
Prep time: 25 min
Cooking time: 7h

Nutrition:
Calories: 200
Points: 4
F: 6g, P: 17g, C: 18g.

Ingredients:
- 3.5lb pork ham hock
- ½ cup vegetable stock
- 1 cup BBQ sauce
- ½ cup peach jam
- ½ cup cherry brandy
- pulled pork seasoning

Recipe:
1. Mix together stock, BBQ, jam, and brandy.
2. Rub the seasoning into the pork, place in Instant Pot.
3. Pour sauce over the top.
4. Cook for 7 hours on Slow Cook.

KOREAN PORK AND PLUM

Serves: 8
Prep time: 5 min
Cooking time: 40 min

Nutrition:
Calories: 315
Points: 8
F: 20g, P: 24g, C: 15g.

Ingredients:
- 2lbs cubed pork belly
- 1 cup bouillon
- 5 ounces tomato passata
- 4 ounces plum jam
- 4 plums, chopped and pitted
- 2 tablespoons hoisin sauce
- 1 tablespoon allspice
- 1 tablespoon cinnamon

Recipe:
1. Rub pork with allspice and cinnamon.
2. Mix remaining ingredients into a sauce.
3. Place pork in Instant Pot, pour the sauce over it.
4. Cook on Stew 40 minutes.

SAUSAGE MEATBALLS

Serves: 8
Prep time: 20 min
Cooking time: 25 min

Nutrition:
Calories: 300
Points: 8
F: 21g, P: 37g, C: 5g.

Ingredients:
- 3lbs Italian sausage
- 2 cups rough toasted crumbs
- 1 cup bone broth
- 1 cup Italian pasta sauce
- 2 eggs
- 3oz mozzarella
- Italian herbs

Recipe:
1. Mix the meat, crumbs, eggs, mozzarella, and seasoning in a bowl.
2. Make into meatballs.
3. Stir and warm the broth and sauce in your Instant Pot until boiling.
4. Gently add the meatballs. Don't let them touch.
5. Seal and cook on Stew 25 minutes.

PORK AND COCONUT CURRY

Serves: 4
Prep time: 20 min
Cooking time: 10 min

Nutrition:
Calories: 450
Points: 10
F: 20g, P: 34g, C: 12g.

Ingredients:
- 2lbs pork shoulder, cubed
- 10oz canned coconut milk
- 2 yellow onions, chopped
- 2 red onions, chopped
- 2 garlic cloves, minced
- 1oz butter sauce
- 2.5tbsp madras paste
- 2tbsp peanut butter

Recipe:
1. Put your Instant Pot on high, add the onions and garlic and soften 5 minutes.
2. Add the pork and stir until browned.
3. Add the remaining ingredients, stir well, seal, cook on Meat for 10 min.
4. Release the pressure slowly.
5. Serve over rice.

CHAR SIU

Serves: 8
Prep time: 5 min
Cooking time: 8h

Nutrition:
Calories: 225
Points: 5
F: 9g, P: 21.5g, C: 13g.

Ingredients:
- 2lbs cubed pork shoulder steak
- ½ cup scallions, chopped
- ½ cup chicken stock
- ¼ cup tamari
- ¼ cup plum sauce
- 3 tablespoons honey
- 3 tablespoons tomato paste, concentrated
- 2 teaspoons minced ginger
- 2 teaspoons minced garlic
- ½ teaspoon 5 spice powder

Recipe:
1. Mix everything but the pork.
2. Place the pork in the slow cooker and pour the sauce over it.
3. Cook for 8 hours on Slow Cook.
4. Depressurise naturally.

PORK PHO

Serves: 6
Prep time: 20 min
Cooking time: 15 min

Nutrition:
Calories: 255
Points: 5
F: 12g, P: 20g, C: 20g.

Ingredients:
- 2lbs lean pork shoulder, minced
- 12oz firm tofu
- 12oz rice noodles
- 1 cup gravy
- 1 cup mixed frozen vegetables
- ¼ cup soy-free Korean stock

Recipe:
1. Put your Instant Pot on high and add the stock and gravy. Heat for 2 min.
2. Add the pork and seal.
3. Cook on Stew for 15 min.
4. Release the pressure quickly, add the noodles and vegetables, seal and cook on Stew for 1 minute.
5. Release the pressure and enjoy.

BBQ PORK LOAF

Serves: 8
Prep time: 15 min
Cooking time: 30 min

Nutrition:
Calories: 340
Points: 8
F: 20g, P: 24g, C: 23g.

Ingredients:
- 3 lbs pork sausage
- 2 cups Panko breadcrumbs
- 1 cup   broth
- ½ cup BBQ sauce
- ½ cup brown sugar
- 4 eggs
- 1tbsp smoked paprika
- 1tbsp cinnamon
- 1tbsp molasses

Recipe:
1. Mix the meat, crumbs, eggs, in one bowl.
2. Put the Steam rack in your Instant Pot and pour in the broth.
3. Mix the BBQ, sugar, paprika, cinnamon, and molasses well.
4. Take some aluminium foil and make a base for your meatloaf with half the mixture on it.
5. Line the base with 1/4 cup BBQ
6. Add the remaining meat and seal into a loaf.
7. Pour the second ¼ cup BBQ on top before wrapping up the foil.
8. Put your meatloaf on your Steam rack.
9. Cook on Steam for 30 min.
10.   Release the pressure quickly and cool.

HAM AND ASPARAGUS STEW

Serves: 6
Prep time: 5 min
Cooking time: 4h

Nutrition:
Calories: 146
Points: 3
F: 6g, P: 15g, C: 5g.

Ingredients:
- 2.5 cups white asparagus
- 1.5 cups lean boiled ham
- 1 cup almond milk
- 2 cups tomato soup
- 2 tablespoons cheddar
- herbes du provence
- salt and pepper to taste

Recipe:
1. Chop the ham and asparagus.
2. Mix all the ingredients in your Instant Pot.
3. Cook on Slow Cook for 4h.

ALMOND MEATBALLS

Serves: 8
Prep time: 15 min
Cooking time: 25 min

Nutrition:
Calories: 370
Points: 9
F: 20g, P: 42g, C: 10g.

Ingredients:
- 3 lbs minced pork shoulder
- 2 cups ground almonds
- 1 cup chicken broth
- 1 cup tomato passata
- 4 eggs
- 3tbsp thyme
- 1tbsp almond oil

Recipe:
1. Mix the meat, almonds, herbs, and eggs in a bowl.
2. Make the meat into balls.
3. Warm the oil in your Instant Pot.
4. Brown the meatballs all over in the oil.
5. Add the broth and sauce.
6. Cook on Stew 25 minutes.

CHEESEBURGER MEATLOAF

Serves: 8
Prep time: 15 min
Cooking time: 30 min

Nutrition:
Calories: 340
Points: 10
F: 21g, P: 27g, C: 23g.

Ingredients:
- 3 lbs 11% fat minced beef
- 2 cups crumbled burger buns
- 1 cup veg broth
- ½ cup cheddar cheese
- ¼ cup American cheese slices
- ¼ cup ketchup
- 4 eggs
- salt and pepper

Recipe:
1. Mix the meat, crumbs, eggs, salt, and pepper, in one bowl.
2. Put the Steam rack in your Instant Pot and pour in the broth.
3. Take some foil and make a base for your meatloaf with half the mixture on it.
4. Line the base with cheddar.
5. Add the remaining meat and seal into a loaf.
6. Dress with ketchup before wrapping in the foil.
7. Put your meatloaf on your Steam rack.
8. Cook on Steam for 30 min.
9. Release the pressure quickly and let your meatloaf cool before serving it.

PORK AND ALE STEW

Serves: 4
Prep time: 5 min
Cooking time: 6h

Nutrition:
Calories: 265
Points: 6
F: 8g, P: 25.5g, C: 20g.

Ingredients:
- 1lb diced pork shoulder
- 1 can tomatoes
- 1 cup diced red onion
- ½ cup beer
- 2 tablespoons honey
- cinnamon
- nutmeg
- salt and pepper

Recipe:
1. Place all ingredients in the Instant Pot.
2. Cook for 6 hours on Slow Cook.

BACON AND SWEET POTATO CASSEROLE

Serves: 6
Prep time: 10 min
Cooking time: 6h

Nutrition:
Calories: 290
Points: 6
F: 10g, P: 12g, C: 40g.

Ingredients:
- 6 rashers bacon, chopped and fried
- 32oz minced sweet potatoes
- 1 cup broth
- 1 cup minced onion
- ½ cup coconut milk
- ½ cup chopped scallions
- salt and pepper

Recipe:
1. Combine everything in your Instant Pot.
2. Cook for 6 hours on Slow Cook.

SWEET AND SPICY PORK

Serves: 8
Prep time: 5 min
Cooking time: 35 min

Nutrition:
Calories: 290
Points: 6
F: 7g, P: 32g, C: 25g.

Ingredients:
- 4lbs diced pork shoulder
- 3 cups diced red onion
- 1 cup fresh lemon and grapefruit, peeled and chopped
- 2/3 cup fresh orange juice
- 1/3 cup sugar-free marmalade
- 2 teaspoons tamarind paste
- 2 teaspoons allspice
- 1 teaspoon aniseed
- 1 teaspoon ginger
- salt and pepper

Recipe:
1. Mix all the ingredients in your Instant Pot.
2. Cook on Meat for 35 minutes.

SCOTCH EGGS

Serves: 8
Prep time: 20 min
Cooking time: 10 min

Nutrition:
Calories: 300
Points: 12
F: 33g, P: 32g, C: 11g.

Ingredients:
- 2lbs sausage
- 8 eggs
- 2 cups almond meal
- 2 tbsp coconut oil
- 1oz mixed herbs
- dipping sauces
- salt and pepper as needed

Recipe:
1. Put the eggs into your Instant Pot and add water to cover, plus half an inch, if your limit allows.
2. Set to Eggs and hard boil.
3. Remove the eggs and put them in ice water.
4. As the eggs chill, split the mince down into 8 balls and flatten them out.
5. Combine the almonds, herbs, and half a tbsp of coconut oil.
6. Once cool, peel the eggs.
7. Place one in each flattened sausage.
8. Roll the sausage into a ball around the egg.
9. Roll in almond meal and coconut oil mix. Sprinkle with salt and pepper.
10. Clear out your Instant Pot and add the remaining oil.
11. Leaving the top open, cook the eggs on high, rolling to ensure even browning.

Lamb

THAI CURRY

Serves: 8
Prep time: 5 min
Cooking time: 45 min

Nutrition:
Calories: 200
Points: 4
F: 5.5g, P: 27.4g, C: 10g.

Ingredients:
- 2lbs chopped lamb, lean
- 2 cups minced red onion
- 1 can coconut milk
- 1 cup beef stock
- ½ cup basil leaves
- 4 minced garlic cloves
- 3 tablespoons curry paste
- 2 tablespoons lime juice
- 1 tablespoons cayenne
- 1 shredded jalapeno pepper
- salt

Recipe:
1. Mix all the ingredients in your Instant Pot.
2. Seal and cook on Stew for 45 minutes.

LAMB ROGAN JOSH

Serves: 6
Prep time: 15 min
Cooking time: 8h

Nutrition:
Calories: 460
Points: 10
F: 28g, P: 38g, C: 14g.

Ingredients:
- 3lbs diced lamb shoulder
- 2 cups minced red onion
- 2 tablespoons thick yoghurt
- 2 tablespoons ghee
- 2 tablespoons lime
- Rogan Josh spice mix
- salt and pepper

Recipe:
1. Mix everything except the yoghurt in your Instant Pot.
2. Cook on Slow Cook for 8h.
3. Serve with yoghurt.

LAMB RAGU

Serves: 6
Prep time: 10 min
Cooking time: 15 min

Nutrition:
Calories: 170
Points: 4
F: 12g, P: 9.5g, C: 6g.

Ingredients:
- 10oz lamb or mutton mince
- 1 can tomato passata
- 1 red onion, diced
- 1 carrot, minced
- 1 garlic clove, minced
- Italian herbs
- salt and pepper

Recipe:
1. Mix all the ingredients in your Instant Pot.
2. Seal and cook on Stew for 15 minutes.

BOBOTIE

Serves: 6
Prep time: 10 min
Cooking time: 25 min

Nutrition:
Calories: 250
Points: 5
F: 7g, P: 28g, C: 15g.

Ingredients:
- 2lbs lean minced lamb
- ¼ cup chopped almonds
- 2 slices stale bread, soaked in milk
- 1 onion chopped
- 5 eggs
- 2tbsp peanut oil
- 1tbsp curry mix
- bay leaves

Recipe:
1. Warm the oil in your Instant Pot.
2. Brown the onions and the minced lamb in the oil.
3. Mix all the remaining ingredients in.
4. Cook for 25 minutes on Stew.

TAGINE

Serves: 6
Prep time: 10 min
Cooking time: 25 min

Nutrition:
Calories: 350
Points: 8
F: 17g, P: 32g, C: 12g.

Ingredients:
- 2lbs lamb shoulder diced
- 1 cup stock
- 2 diced onions
- 3.5oz almond slivers
- Moroccan spices
- rose petals
- 3tbsp olive oil
- 2 cups rice, to serve

Recipe:
1. Mix 2tbsp of the oil with the spices and rub into the lamb.
2. Heat 1tbso of the oil in your Instant Pot.
3. Add the onion and cook it for five minutes.
4. Add the lamb and brown all over.
5. Add the remaining ingredients, seal, and cook 25 minutes on Stew.
6. Release the pressure slowly and serve over rice.

LAMB CARNITAS

Serves: 8
Prep time: 15 min
Cooking time: 40 min

Nutrition:
Calories: 230
Points: 5
F: 7g, P: 27g, C: 5g.

Ingredients:
- 2lbs diced lamb shank
- ½ cup mint sauce
- ½ cup red wine
- ½ cup orange juice
- juice of one lime
- juice of one lemon
- 1 tablespoon olive oil

Recipe:
1. Rub the chicken with the mint sauce
2. Put in Instant Pot. Pour wine and juices on top.
3. Cook on Stew for 40 min.
4. Remove and shred.

ITALIAN LAMB

Serves: 8
Prep time: 5 min
Cooking time: 15 min

Nutrition:
Calories: 265
Points: 6
F: 14g, P: 20g, C: 3g.

Ingredients:
- 2lbs diced lamb shoulder
- 3.50z cherry tomatoes
- 3.50z black and green olives, pitted
- ½ cup white wine
- juice of 3 lemons
- Italian herbs
- 4tbsp olive oil
- salt and pepper
- couscous, to serve

Recipe:
1. Mix all the ingredients.
2. Seal your Instant Pot and cook 15 minutes on Stew.

LAMB AND KALE BAKE

Serves: 8
Prep time: 5 min
Cooking time: 40 min

Nutrition:
Calories: 275
Points: 6
F: 9g, P: 28g, C: 20g.

Ingredients:
- 24 ounces of diced stewing lamb
- 12 ounces of kale
- 1 can evaporated milk, low fat
- 1 can mushroom soup
- 1 cup greek yoghurt
- ¼ cup red wine
- ¼ cup flour
- dash of Worcestershire sauce
- salt and pepper

Recipe:
1. Mix the liquids and seasonings into a sauce.
2. Put the chicken and broccoli into the slow cooker. Pour the sauce on top.
3. Cook on Stew for 40 minutes.

LAMB MEATLOAF

Serves: 6
Prep time: 10 min
Cooking time: 25 min

Nutrition:
Calories: 300
Points: 6
F: 16g, P: 32g, C: 5g.

Ingredients:
- 1.5lb lamb mince
- 1.5 cups diced onion
- 2 eggs
- ¼ cup minced garlic
- 2 tablespoons mint sauce
- 2 teaspoons mustard
- 1 teaspoon Italian herbs
- salt and pepper

Recipe:
1. Combine lamb, eggs, onion, garlic, herbs, and salt and pepper.
2. Form a loaf and place on some foil and into slow cooker.
3. Mix mint, mustard, and salt and pepper.
4. Spread mint mix over the loaf.
5. Cook on low for 5 hours.

RED WINE LAMB STEW

Serves: 4
Prep time: 5 min
Cooking time: 40 min

Nutrition:
Calories: 268
Points: 5
F: 8g, P: 25.5g, C: 21g.

Ingredients:
- 1lb boneless, fat-trimmed, lamb shoulder, cubed
- 1 can tomatoes
- 1 cup diced onion
- ½ cup red wine
- 1 tablespoon honey
- 1 tablespoon minced garlic
- herbes de provence
- salt and pepper

Recipe:
1. Put all the ingredients in your Instant Pot.
2. Cook on Stew 40 minutes.

LAMB HASH BROWN CASSEROLE

Serves: 6
Prep time: 10 min
Cooking time: 6h

Nutrition:
Calories: 290
Points: 6
F: 10g, P: 12g, C: 40g.

Ingredients:
- 12oz lamb mince
- 32oz grated potatoes
- 1 cup bone broth
- 1 cup chopped onion
- ½ cup chopped scallions
- salt and pepper

Recipe:
1. Combine everything in your Instant Pot.
2. Set to Slow Cook and cook for 6 hours.

LAMB AND APRICOTS

Serves: 12
Prep time: 30 min
Cooking time: 40 min

Nutrition:
Calories: 200
Points: 4
F: 6g, P: 17g, C: 18g.

Ingredients:
- 3.5lb lamb shoulder
- ½ cup beef stock
- 1 cup BBQ sauce
- ½ cup apricot jam
- ½ cup fresh apricots
- ½ cup brandy

Recipe:
1. Mix together stock, BBQ, jam, and apricots.
2. Slice top of lamb and place in Instant Pot.
3. Pour sauce over the top.
4. Cook on Stew for 40 minutes.

LAMB CHAR SIU

Serves: 8
Prep time: 5 min
Cooking time: 8h

Nutrition:
Calories: 230
Points: 6
F: 9g, P: 21.5g, C: 12.7g.

Ingredients:
- 2lbs lamb, chopped
- ½ cup vegetable broth
- ¼ cup soy sauce
- ¼ cup hoisin sauce
- 3 tablespoons sugar
- 2 teaspoons minced garlic
- 2 teaspoons minced ginger
- ½ teaspoon 5 spice powder

Recipe:
1. Mix all the seasonings.
2. Place lamb in Instant Pot and pour sauce on top.
3. Cook for 8 hours on Slow Cook.

ROSEMARY LAMB

Serves: 6
Prep time: 10 min
Cooking time: 25 min

Nutrition:
Calories: 225
Points: 8
F: 16g, P: 25g, C: 5g.

Ingredients:
- 3lbs lamb mince
- 2 cups stock
- 1 cup red wine
- 2 carrots diced
- 2 celery stalks diced
- 1 onion diced
- 2tbsp rosemary, dry
- 1tbsp olive oil
- salt and pepper

Recipe:
1. Heat the oil in your Instant Pot.
2. Brown the lamb.
3. Add the onion and cook until softened.
4. Add the remaining ingredients and mix well.
5. Seal and cook on Stew 25 minutes.
6. Depressurize naturally.

LAMB CHILI

Serves: 8
Prep time: 5 min
Cooking time: 50 min

Nutrition:
Calories: 210
Points: 4
F: 8g, P: 21g, C: 11g.

Ingredients:
- 1.5lbs lamb mince
- 2 cans tomatoes
- 2 cups diced red onion
- 1 cup diced red pepper
- 1 cup stock
- 2 ounces dark chocolate
- 2 teaspoons minced garlic
- chili mix

Recipe:
1. Put the oil in your Instant Pot and warm.
2. Put the onions in your Instant Pot and soften 5 minutes.
3. Add the remaining ingredients and cook on Stew 50 minutes.

Seafood

SALMON LAKSA

Serves: 4
Prep time: 5 min
Cooking time: 30 min

Nutrition:
Calories: 700
Points: 16
F: 39g, P: 46g, C: 44g.

Ingredients:
- 4 salmon fillets
- 1 cup bouillon
- 1 can coconut milk
- 1 zucchini, shredded
- 1 cup bean sprouts
- 200g vermicelli noodles
- a jar of laksa paste

Recipe:
1. Mix all the ingredients except the noodles.
2. Cook on Stew for 30 minutes.
3. Depressurize quickly and stir in the noodles.
4. When the noodles are soft, serve.

SHRIMP AND COCONUT SOUP

Serves: 4
Prep time: 5 min
Cooking time: 8 min

Nutrition:
Calories: 185
Points: 4
F: 6g, P: 21g, C: 12g.

Ingredients:
- 1lb prepped shrimp
- 1.5 cups vegetable bouillon
- 1 can coconut milk
- 1 cup diced red and yellow peppers
- 1 tablespoon osyter sauce
- 1 tablespoon lime juice

Recipe:
1. Mix all the ingredients.
2. Cook on Fish for 8 minutes.

SWEET AND HOT LEMON SHRIMP

Serves: 4
Prep time: 7 min
Cooking time: 8 min

Nutrition:
Calories: 180
Points: 3
F: 5g, P: 28g, C: 3g.

Ingredients:
- 1.5lbs peeled and deveined shrimp
- 2/3 cup of cream
- 1 cup minced mixed vegetables
- 1 chile
- 1 tablespoon lemon zest
- 1 tablespoon lemon juice
- 1 tablespoon sugar
- salt and pepper

Recipe:
1. Blend the chile, cream, sugar, lemon and salt and pepper.
2. Put in your Instant Pot, add the shrimp and vegetables and cook on Stew for 8 minutes.

COD PHO

Serves: 6
Prep time: 10 min
Cooking time: 17 min

Nutrition:
Calories: 200
Points: 3
F: 3g, P: 20g, C: 8g.

Ingredients:
- 2lbs skinless, boneless cod
- 12oz zucchini, spiralized
- 1 cup fish stock
- ¼ cup soy-free Korean stock
- ¼ cup oyster sauce

Recipe:
1. Put your Instant Pot on high and add the stocks. Cook for 2 min.
2. Add the cod and seal.
3. Cook on Fish for 15 min.
4. Release the pressure quickly, add the zucchini, seal and cook on Stew for 1 more min.
5. Release the pressure and serve hot.

MUSTARD KING PRAWNS

Serves: 4
Prep time: 10 min
Cooking time: 5 min

Nutrition:
Calories: 180
Points: 3
F: 5g, P: 23g, C: 9g.

Ingredients:
- 1lb jumbo prawns
- 1 cup orange puree
- 1 cup diced scallions
- ¼ cup cilantro
- 1 tablespoon hot sauce
- 1 tablespoon mustard
- 1 tablespoon lime juice

Recipe:
1. Mix all the ingredients together in the Instant Pot.
2. Cook on Fish for 5 minutes.

GINGER SHRIMP

Serves: 4
Prep time: 5 min
Cooking time: 5 min

Nutrition:
Calories: 185
Points: 4
F: 6g, P: 24g, C: 5g.

Ingredients:
- 1lb prepped shrimp
- 1 cup minced onion
- 1 cup minced garlic
- ½ cup water
- 1 tablespoon mirin
- 2 teaspoons tamari
- 1 teaspoon fresh ginger, grated finely
- 1 teaspoon tahini
- 1 teaspoon sugar
- salt and pepper

Recipe:
1. Mix all the ingredients together in your Instant Pot.
2. Seal and cook on Stew for 5 minutes.

CATFISH AND BEANSPROUTS

Serves: 5
Prep time: 10 min
Cooking time: 25 min

Nutrition:
Calories: 120
Points: 2
F: 4g, P: 28g, C: 10g.

Ingredients:
- 2lbs prepped catfish
- 20oz fish stock
- 2 cups beansprouts
- 1 shredded onion
- 4 garlic cloves, minced
- 4tbsp oyster sauce
- 2tbsp soya sauce

Recipe:
1. Mix all the ingredients in your Instant Pot.
2. Set to Stew and cook for 25 minutes.
3. Release the pressure quickly and serve over rice.

HAKE AND SQUASH SOUP

Serves: 4
Prep time: 10 min
Cooking time: 8h

Nutrition:
Calories: 335
Points: 7
F: 8g, P: 35g, C: 22g.

Ingredients:
- 1.5lbs prepared hake
- 3 cups bouillon
- ½lb pumpkin puree
- ½ lb chopped butternut squash
- ½ tin coconut milk
- thai red curry paste

Recipe:
1. Mix the sauce.
2. Put the fish in the Instant Pot and pour the sauce over it.
3. Cook on Slow Cook for 8h.

SPICY HORSERADISH SHRIMP

Serves: 4
Prep time: 5 min
Cooking time: 5 min

Nutrition:
Calories: 150
Points: 4
F: 3g, P: 25g, C: 9g.

Ingredients:
- 1lb peeled and deveined shrimp
- 1 cup diced green onion
- ¼ cup cilantro, fresh
- 1 tablespoon horseradish
- 1 tablespoon hot chilli sauce
- 1 tablespoon lime juice

Recipe:
1. Mix everything in your Instant Pot.
2. Cook on Fish for 5 minutes.

PULPO CON CHILE

Serves: 4
Prep time: 5 min
Cooking time: 30 min

Nutrition:
Calories: 120
Points: 2
F: 0g, P: 21g, C: 5g.

Ingredients:
- 2lbs octopus, chopped
- 1 cup tomato puree
- 1 onion, minced
- 3 cloves garlic, minced
- 3tbsp smoked paprika
- 1tbsp ghost chili sauce
- salt and pepper

Recipe:
1. Mix all the ingredients in your Instant Pot.
2. Seal and cook on Meat for 30 minutes.

CHILAQUILES

Serves: 10
Prep time: 15 min
Cooking time: 35 min

Nutrition:
Calories: 220
Points: 4
F: 2g, P: 24g, C: 23g.

Ingredients:
- 2.5lbs boneless cod, chopped
- 5 cups plain or salted tortilla chips
- 2 cans chopped tomatoes
- 2 cups chopped green bell peppers
- 2 cups chopped red onion
- 1 cup chopped chiles
- ¾ cup bouillon
- 2/3 cup queso fresco
- ¼ cup cilantro, fresh

Recipe:
1. Mix everything except the tortilla chips and cheese, into the Instant Pot.
2. Cook on Fish for 35 minutes.
3. Depressurize quickly.
4. Layer tortilla chips on top and crumble cheese all over.

GARLIC SQUID

Serves: 4
Prep time: 5 min
Cooking time: 25 min

Nutrition:
Calories: 105
Points: 1
F: 1g, P: 21g, C: 2g.

Ingredients:
- 2lb squid, diced
- 1 white onion, minced
- 3 cloves garlic, minced
- salt and pepper to taste
- olive oil

Recipe:
1. Put the oil in the base of your Instant Pot and set to high.
2. Soften the onion in it for 5 minutes.
3. Add the garlic and cook another minute.
4. Add the remaining ingredients and enough water to cover it all.
5. Cook on Stew for 25 minutes.

CRAB RAGU

Serves: 6
Prep time: 10 min
Cooking time: 10 min

Nutrition:
Calories: 105
Points: 2
F: 4.5g, P: 14g, C: 3g.

Ingredients:
- 10oz fresh crab meat
- 1 cup fish stock
- 1 onion, diced
- 1 garlic clove, minced
- 1tbsp sage
- 1tbsp fennel
- salt and pepper

Recipe:
1. Mix all the ingredients in your Instant Pot.
2. Seal and cook on Fish for 10 minutes.

SALMON AND POTATOES

Serves: 4
Prep time: 5 min
Cooking time: 2h

Nutrition:
Calories: 160
Points: 7
F: 20g, P: 34g, C: 11g.

Ingredients:
- 4 skinless salmon fillets
- 2 oz whole baby potatoes
- 1oz cherry tomatoes
- juice of one lemon
- 2 tablespoons thyme
- salt and pepper

Recipe:
1. Rub the salmon with salt, pepper, lemon juice, and thyme.
2. Place in the Instant Pot with potatoes, tomatoes, and the minimum water.
3. Cook on Slow Cook for 2h.

MUSSELS WITH GARLIC

Serves: 4
Prep time: 6 min
Cooking time: 1 min

Nutrition:
Calories: 130
Points: 2
F: 3g, P: 22g, C: 1g.

Ingredients:
- 2lbs whole mussels
- 1 cup dry white wine
- 1 minced white onion
- 1tsp olive oil
- 1tsp minced garlic

Recipe:
1. Clean the mussels.
2. Put the mussels in the steamer basket.
3. Cook the onion in the olive oil 5 minutes.
4. Add the water, wine, and garlic.
5. Put the steamer basket in the cooker, bring to pressure and cook for one minute.
6. Discard any unopened mussels.
7. Serve with the garlic-wine sauce on top.

Vegetarian & Vegan

VEGAN CONGEE - SWEET

Serves: 6
Prep time: 10 min
Cooking time: 25 min

Nutrition:
Calories: 104
Points: 2
F: 2g, P: 2g, C: 22g.

Ingredients:
- 6 cups warmed soya or almond milk
- 1 cup uncooked Arborio rice
- 1 cup diced mango
- 1 cup diced apple
- 1 teaspoon cinnamon powder
- 1 teaspoon grated fresh ginger
- 1 teaspoon salt

Recipe:
1. Mix the ingredients in your Instant Pot.
2. Seal and cook on Rice.
3. Release the pressure naturally.

VEGAN CONGEE - SAVORY

Serves: 6
Prep time: 10 min
Cooking time: 25 min

Nutrition:
Calories: 184
Points: 4
F: 7g, P: 11g, C: 22g.

Ingredients:
- 6 cups warmed vegetable broth
- 1 cup uncooked Arborio rice
- 3 cups chopped fried tofu
- 1 yellow onion, chopped
- 2 scallions, chopped
- 1 teaspoon soy sauce
- 1 teaspoon salt

Recipe:
1. Mix the ingredients in your Instant Pot.
2. Seal and cook on Rice.
3. Release the pressure naturally.

VEGAN CONGEE – SOY-FREE

Serves: 6
Prep time: 10 min
Cooking time: 25 min

Nutrition:
Calories: 114
Points: 2
F: 2g, P: 2g, C: 24g.

Ingredients:
- 6 cups warmed vegetable broth
- 1 cup uncooked Arborio rice
- 2 cups shiitake mushrooms
- 1 cup chopped bamboo
- 1 minced red onion
- 1 teaspoon grated fresh ginger
- 1 teaspoon salt

Recipe:
1. Mix the ingredients in your Instant Pot.
2. Seal and cook on Rice.
3. Release the pressure naturally.

VEGGIE-SAUSAGE SCRAMBLE

Serves: 6
Prep time: 5 min
Cooking time: 15 min

Nutrition:
Calories: 360
Points: 8
F: 16g, P: 21g, C: 44g.

Ingredients:
- 1 pound firm tofu
- 6 cups cubed chapatti bread
- 2 cups sliced mushrooms
- 2 cups crumbled cooked vegan sausage
- 1½ cups plain almond milk
- 1 medium-size yellow onion, minced
- 3 garlic cloves, minced
- 2 teaspoons olive oil
- ¼ teaspoon red pepper flakes
- 3 tablespoons nutritional yeast
- Salt and pepper

Recipe:
1. Crumble the tofu and pat it dry with a clean cloth.
2. Warm the oil in your Instant Pot and cook the onion 5 minutes.
3. Add the garlic, mushrooms, cook another 2 minutes.
4. Add the spices.
5. Pulse the tofu, milk, and nutritional yeast.
6. Put the bread in your Instant Pot, add sausage and vegetables.
7. Pour the tofu in.
8. Seal and cook on Stew for 15 minutes.

VEGAN ARTICHOKE OMELET

Serves: 4
Prep time: 10 min
Cooking time: 15 min

Nutrition:
Calories: 250
Points: 5
F: 6g, P: 23g, C: 14g.

Ingredients:
- 1lb drained tofu, firm
- 2 cups canned or thawed frozen artichoke hearts, chopped
- 5 scallions, diced
- ½ cup chopped sun-dried tomatoes
- 3 tablespoons nutritional yeast
- 1 tablespoon cornstarch
- 2 teaspoons olive oil
- ½ teaspoon dried thyme
- ½ teaspoon onion powder
- ½ teaspoon dried basil
- Salt and pepper

Recipe:
1. Blend the tofu, nutritional yeast, cornstarch, onion powder, salt and pepper with a few tomatoes.
2. Warm the oil in the base of your Instant Pot.
3. Add the scallions, herbs, remaining tomatoes, and some salt and pepper and cook 5 minutes.
4. Stir the tofu into the veg.
5. Seal and cook on Stew for 15 minutes.
6. Remove and cut into slices.

VEGAN POTATO OMELET

Serves: 4
Prep time: 10 min
Cooking time: 15 min

Nutrition:
Calories: 322
Points: 7
F: 6g, P: 23g, C: 34g.

Ingredients:
- 1lb drained tofu, firm
- 2 cups potatoes, part cooked
- 1 cup chopped red peppers
- ½ cup chopped mushrooms
- ½ cup chopped onions
- 3 tablespoons nutritional yeast
- 1 tablespoon cornstarch
- 2 teaspoons olive oil
- ½ teaspoon smoked paprika
- ½ teaspoon cayenne pepper
- ½ teaspoon onion powder
- Salt and pepper

Recipe:
1. Blend the tofu, nutritional yeast, cornstarch, onion powder, salt and pepper.
2. Warm the oil in the base of your Instant Pot.
3. Add the vegetables, herbs, and some salt and pepper and cook 5 minutes.
4. Stir the tofu into the veg.
5. Seal and cook on Stew for 15 minutes.
6. Remove and cut into slices.

VEGAN OLIVE OMELET

Serves: 4
Prep time: 10 min
Cooking time: 15 min

Nutrition:
Calories: 277
Points: 6
F: 9g, P: 23g, C: 14g.

Ingredients:
- 1lb drained tofu, firm
- 2 cups chopped mushrooms
- 1 cup minced onion
- ½ cup chopped black olives
- 3 tablespoons nutritional yeast
- 1 tablespoon cornstarch
- 2 teaspoons olive oil
- ½ teaspoon lemon juice
- ½ teaspoon tomato puree
- ½ teaspoon onion powder
- Salt and pepper

Recipe:
1. Blend the tofu, nutritional yeast, cornstarch, onion powder, salt and pepper.
2. Warm the oil in the base of your Instant Pot.
3. Add the vegetables, tomato, lemon juice, and some salt and pepper and cook 5 minutes.
4. Stir the tofu into the veg.
5. Seal and cook on Stew for 15 minutes.
6. Remove and cut into slices.
7. Serve with vegan feta.

MUSHROOM OMELET

Serves: 4
Prep time: 10 min
Cooking time: 15 min

Nutrition:
Calories: 320
Points: 7
F: 8g, P: 26g, C: 11g.

Ingredients:
- 6 eggs
- 2 cups white mushrooms, chopped
- 1 cup shiitake mushrooms, chopped
- 1 cup wild mushrooms, chopped
- ½ cup milk
- 2 teaspoons olive oil
- ½ teaspoon paprika
- ½ teaspoon garlic powder
- ½ teaspoon onion powder
- Salt and pepper

Recipe:
1. Whisk the eggs with milk, salt, pepper, paprika, garlic powder, and onion powder.
2. Warm the oil in the base of your Instant Pot.
3. Add the mushrooms and some salt and pepper and cook 5 minutes.
4. Stir the eggs into the mushrooms.
5. Seal and cook on Stew for 15 minutes.
6. Remove and cut into slices.

TORTILLA CON CEBOLLA

Serves: 4
Prep time: 10 min
Cooking time: 15 min

Nutrition:
Calories: 314
Points: 6
F: 8g, P: 27g, C: 33g.

Ingredients:
- 6 eggs
- 2 cups part cooked white potatoes, cubed
- 1 cup sliced white onion
- ½ cup minced garlic
- 2 teaspoons olive oil
- ½ teaspoon paprika
- ½ teaspoon nutmeg
- ½ teaspoon onion powder
- Salt and pepper

Recipe:
1. Whisk the eggs with salt, pepper, paprika, nutmeg, and onion powder.
2. Warm the oil in the base of your Instant Pot.
3. Add the potato, onion, garlic, and some salt and pepper and cook 5 minutes.
4. Stir the eggs into the veg.
5. Seal and cook on Stew for 15 minutes.
6. Remove and cut into slices.

CHEESY OMELET

Serves: 4
Prep time: 10 min
Cooking time: 15 min

Nutrition:
Calories: 344
Points: 9
F: 12g, P: 32g, C: 13g.

Ingredients:
- 6 eggs
- 2 cups shredded cheddar
- ½ cup chopped red onion
- 2 teaspoons olive oil
- ½ teaspoon cayenne
- ½ teaspoon onion powder
- Salt and pepper

Recipe:
1. Whisk the eggs with salt, pepper, and onion powder.
2. Warm the oil in the base of your Instant Pot.
3. Add the onion, and some salt and pepper and cook 5 minutes.
4. Stir the eggs into the onion.
5. Sprinkle with cheddar.
6. Seal and cook on Stew for 15 minutes.
7. Remove and cut into slices.

TEMPEH AND LENTILS

Serves: 4
Prep time: 5 min
Cooking time: 30 min

Nutrition:
Calories: 320
Points: 6
F: 7g, P: 13g, C: 50g.

Ingredients:
- 8oz tempeh
- 3 cups cooked lentils
- 1 can chopped tomato
- 1.5 cups vegetable broth
- 1 cup diced cauliflower
- 1 cup chopped dry fruit
- 1 spring onion, minced
- 3 minced garlic cloves
- 2tsp olive oil
- ½ tsp cumin
- ¼ tsp cinnamon
- ¼ tsp cayenne
- salt and pepper

Recipe:
1. Put your Instant Pot on high and add the oil.
2. When the oil is hot add the onion and soften it for 5 minutes.
3. Add in the garlic, tomato, cumin, cinnamon, cayenne, and stir for a minute to mix.
4. Add the broth, tempeh, lentils, tomatoes, fruit, cauliflower, salt and pepper. Cook on Stew for 30 minutes.

QUINOA STUFFED BELL PEPPERS

Serves: 4
Prep time: 10 min
Cooking time: 25 min

Nutrition:
Calories: 230
Points: 4
F: 4g, P: 11g, C: 27g.

Ingredients:
- 4 large bell peppers, hollowed
- 2 cups cooked quinoa
- 1 cup baby green peas
- ½ cup chopped parsley
- ⅓ cup minced sun-dried tomatoes
- 1 jar marinated artichoke hearts, drained and chopped
- 1 large red onion, minced
- 2 teaspoons olive oil
- 2 teaspoons freshly squeezed lemon juice
- ½ teaspoon dried marjoram
- Salt and pepper

Recipe:
1. Warm the oil in your Instant Pot.
2. When hot, add the onion and soften for 5 minutes.
3. Add the tomatoes and marjoram.
4. Put the mix in a bowl and add the quinoa, artichokes, peas, parsley, lemon, and salt and pepper.
5. Divide the stuffing between the peppers and put them in the steamer basket of your Instant Pot.
6. Put a cup of water in your Instant Pot.
7. Insert the steamer basket.
8. Seal and cook on Steam for 25 minutes.
9. Depressurize naturally and serve immediately.

CORN ON THE COB

Serves: 4
Prep time: 10 min
Cooking time: 19 min

Nutrition:
Calories: 300
Points: 6
F: 3.5g, P: 4.5g, C: 32g.

Ingredients:
- 8 ears corn
- 1 cup hot water
- herbs or paprika
- olive spread

Recipe:
1. Cut the ears of corn to fit the steamer basket in your Instant Pot.
2. Put the ears of corn, surrounded by herbs or dusted with paprika, in your steamer basket.
3. Pour the water in your Instant Pot and lower the basket into it.
4. Seal and cook on Steam for 18 minutes.
5. Depressurize quickly, top with olive spread and serve.

ELOTES

Serves: 4
Prep time: 10 min
Cooking time: 19 min

Nutrition:
Calories: 300
Points: 7
F: 10g, P: 9g, C: 32g.

Ingredients:
- 8 ears corn
- 1 cup hot water
- 1 cup cream cheese
- ½ cup mixed shredded cheese
- ½ cup breadcrumbs
- 2tbsp paprika
- olive spread

Recipe:
1. Cut the ears of corn to fit the steamer basket in your Instant Pot.
2. Put the ears of corn, surrounded by herbs or dusted with paprika, in your steamer basket.
3. Pour the water in your Instant Pot and lower the basket into it.
4. Seal and cook on Steam for 18 minutes.
5. Depressurize quickly, top with olive spread and dip in breadcrumbs.
6. Spread cream cheese all over.
7. Sprinkle with shredded cheese.
8. Eat when the cheese starts melting in.

SEITAN ROAST

Serves: 8
Prep time: 15 min
Cooking time: 30 min

Nutrition:
Calories:
Points:
F: g, P: g, C: g.

Ingredients:
- 2lbs seitan
- 10oz spinach
- 1 vegan sausage, chopped
- 3 red onions, minced
- 3 garlic cloves, minced
- 2 cups mushrooms, minced
- 1 roasted red bell pepper, minced
- ½ teaspoon dried thyme
- ½ teaspoon dried crumbled sage
- 2 teaspoons olive oil
- salt and pepper

Recipe:
1. Warm the oil in the base of your Instant Pot.
2. Add the onion and soften for 5 minutes.
3. Add the garlic, mushrooms, herbs. Cook for another 2 minutes.
4. Add the spinach, bell pepper, and a little salt and pepper. Cook for another 2 minutes.
5. Remove from the heat.
6. Mix with the sausage and put aside for later.
7. Roll your seitan out onto some aluminium foil.
8. Spread the stuffing evenly on your seitan and roll it up.
9. Use the foil to seal it. Place in your Instant Pot steamer basket.
10. Put hot water in your Instant Pot and lower the steamer basket.
11. Cook on Steam for 30 minutes.
12. Depressurize naturally.

Soups

PEA AND HAM SOUP

Serves: 6
Prep time: 5 min
Cooking time: 5 min

Nutrition:
Calories: 170
Points: 4
F: 6g, P: 9g, C: 18g.

Ingredients:
- 6 cups water
- 3.5oz diced ham hock
- 2 cups dry green peas
- 1 carrot diced
- 1 onion diced
- 1 celery stalk diced
- 1tbsp butter
- salt and pepper

Recipe:
1. Put the butter, ham, and onion in the pressure cooker on high heat and stir until browned.
2. Add all the other ingredients. Make sure it's only ½ full.
3. Stir well and seal.
4. Put on high and cook for 5 minutes.

CHICKEN NOODLE SOUP

Serves: 4
Prep time: 5 min
Cooking time: 8 min

Nutrition:
Calories: 120
Points: 3
F: 5g, P: 6g, C: 16g.

Ingredients:
- 4 cups chicken or vegetable stock
- 1 cup diced chicken
- 6oz dry noodles
- 1 cup diced onion
- 1 cup diced celery
- 1 cup diced carrots
- 1 cup diced red bell pepper

Recipe:
1. Put all the ingredients in your Instant Pot.
2. Seal and cook on Stew for 8 minutes.

COFFEE AND PORK STEW

Serves: 6
Prep time: 10 min
Cooking time: 25 min

Nutrition:
Calories: 400
Points: 9
F: 20g, P: 37g, C: 4g.

Ingredients:
- 2.5 lbs diced pork shoulder
- 3 cups strong coffee
- 1 cup bone broth
- 1 cup red wine
- 1 minced onion
- 3tbsp olive oil
- 2tbsp garlic
- salt, pepper

Recipe:
1. Put the oil in the Instant Pot and soften the onion for 5 minutes.
2. Add the pork and brown.
3. Add the remaining ingredients.
4. Seal and cook on Stew 25 minutes.

PUMPKIN SPICE SOUP

Serves: 3
Prep time: 10 min
Cooking time: 10 min

Nutrition:
Calories: 130
Points: 2
F: 2g, P: 13g, C: 7g.

Ingredients:
- 2 cups pumpkin puree
- 1.5 cups chicken broth
- 2 tablespoons butter
- 1 minced onion
- 2 cloves roasted garlic, minced
- 4 slices cooked bacon
- ½ teaspoon ginger
- ¼ teaspoon cinnamon
- ¼ teaspoon coriander
- 1/8 teaspoon nutmeg
- salt and pepper

Recipe:
1. Melt the butter in your Instant Pot.
2. When hot, add the onion, ginger, and garlic and soften 3 minutes.
3. Add the remaining ingredients.
4. Seal and cook on Stew 10 minutes.
5. Depressurize naturally.
6. Blend.

BEEF AND BROCCOLI SOUP

Serves: 4
Prep time: 10 min
Cooking time: 40 min

Nutrition:
Calories: 430
Points: 10
F: 17g, P: 54g, C: 4g.

Ingredients:
- 2lbs stewing steak, finely chopped
- 1lb broccoli, chopped
- 1 cup bone broth
- 3 garlic cloves, minced
- 1tsp ginger
- 1tsp olive oil
- ½ tsp chili flakes
- salt and pepper

Recipe:
1. Mix all the ingredients in your Instant Pot.
2. Seal and cook on Stew for 40 minutes.
3. Depressurize naturally.
4. Remove the beef.
5. Blend the sauce.
6. Add the beef back in.

CHICKEN CHOWDER

Serves: 4
Prep time: 15 min
Cooking time: 25 min

Nutrition:
Calories: 355
Points: 11
F: 28g, P: 21g, C: 6g.

Ingredients:
- 1/2lb chicken meat, lean, cubed
- 1/2lb bacon
- 1 cup chicken stock
- 1/2 cup heavy cream
- 1 minced onion
- 1 sliced leek
- 1 stalk celery, diced
- 2tbsp butter
- 1tsp thyme
- salt and pepper

Recipe:
1. Put 1tbsp of butter in the Instant Pot and heat it.
2. Add the onion, celery, and leek and soften.
3. Add the remaining butter, the spices and chicken and brown everything.
4. Add the bacon, stock, and cream.
5. Seal and cook on Stew 25 minutes.

COD STEW

Serves: 7
Prep time: 10 min
Cooking time: 10 min

Nutrition:
Calories: 135
Points: 2
F: 3g, P: 19g, C: 5g.

Ingredients:
- 4 cups fish stock
- 2 cups lean cod, diced
- 2 cups spinach
- 4 rashers bacon, chopped
- 1 onion, chopped
- 1 cup celery, chopped
- 1 cup courgette, chopped
- ¼ cup fresh chopped coriander leaf
- 1tbsp olive oil
- salt and pepper

Recipe:
1. Fry the bacon in your Instant Pot for 2 minutes.
2. Add the onions and soften 5 minutes.
3. Add the remaining ingredients and seal.
4. Cook on Stew for 10 minutes.

PIZZA STEW

Serves: 8
Prep time: 5 min
Cooking time: 25 min

Nutrition:
Calories: 450
Points: 10
F: 18g, P: 15g, C: 18g.

Ingredients:
- 1lb chopped ham
- 1lb chopped potatoes
- 2 cups chopped tomatoes
- 6oz mozzarella cubes
- 2oz pepperoni
- 1tbsp onion powder
- 1tbsp Italian herbs
- 1tsp garlic powder

Recipe:
1. Put all the ingredients except the cheese in the Instant Pot.
2. Seal and cook on Stew 25 minutes.
3. Depressurize and top with cheese before serving.

HERBY SOUP

Serves: 6
Prep time: 5 min
Cooking time: 25 min

Nutrition:
Calories: 80
Points: 1
F: 1g, P: 4g, C: 16g.

Ingredients:
- 1 cup white wine
- 2 cups vegetable stock
- 2 carrots diced
- 2 celery stalks diced
- 1 sweet potato diced
- 1 onion diced
- 2tbsp rosemary
- 2tbsp thyme
- 2tbsp sage
- 1tbsp garlic paste
- salt and pepper

Recipe:
1. Mix all the ingredients in your Instant Pot.
2. Seal and cook on Stew for 25 minutes.
3. Release the pressure naturally.
4. Blend.

Green Bean Stew

Serves: 6
Prep time: 10 min
Cooking time: 5 min

Nutrition:
Calories: 55
Points: 1
F: 3g, P: 2g, C: 6g.

Ingredients:
- 1lb green beans
- 2 cups chopped tomatoes
- 1 diced onion
- 1 tbsp minced garlic
- 1tbsp olive oil
- Italian herbs
- salt and pepper

Recipe:
1. Trim your beans and cut them around two inches long.
2. Use oil to add some colour to the beans and onion.
3. Add the remaining ingredients and use water to make up to your minimum fluid amount.
4. Cook on Stew for 5 minutes.

CLAM CHOWDER

Serves: 6
Prep time: 5 min
Cooking time: 20 min

Nutrition:
Calories: 400
Points: 16
F: 35g, P: 22g, C: 12g.

Ingredients:
- 22oz clams in juice
- 2 cups cubed belly bacon
- 2 cups milk
- 1 cup cream
- 1 cup white wine
- 4 peeled and chopped medium potatoes
- 2 chopped onions
- 4tbsp Provence herbs
- 2tbsp butter
- 2tbsp flour
- salt and pepper

Recipe:
1. Put your bacon in your Instant Pot on low, to get the fat to melt a bit.
2. Add the onion and potatoes to soften and brown.
3. Add the wine and stir well.
4. Mix the butter and flour to form a thick paste. Dissolve in the wine.
5. Add the milk.
6. When the sauce is thick, add the remaining ingredients.
7. Cook for 15 minutes on Stew.
8. Depressurize naturally.

WILD RICE SOUP

Serves: 4
Prep time: 5 min
Cooking time: 12 min

Nutrition:
Calories: 200
Points:
F: 1g, P: 5g, C: 42g.

Ingredients:
- 4 cups chicken stock
- 2 cups cooked wild rice
- 20 diced white mushrooms
- 2 diced celery sticks
- 1 diced carrot
- 1 diced onion
- salt and pepper

Recipe:
1. Put all the ingredients in your Instant Pot and seal.
2. Cook 12 minutes on Stew.

Black Bean Stew

Serves: 6
Prep time: 5 min
Cooking time: 20 min

Nutrition:
Calories: 280
Points: 5
F: 2g, P: 17g, C: 50g.

Ingredients:
- 1lb black beans, rinsed and soaked overnight
- 4 cups chicken stock
- 2 chopped onions
- 2 diced carrots
- ¼ cup fresh cilantro
- 3tbsp herb mix
- 2tbsp lime juice
- 1tbsp chili paste
- salt and pepper

Recipe:
1. Mix all ingredients in the Instant Pot.
2. Put the lid on and cook on Stew for 20 minutes.

Crab Soup

Serves: 6
Prep time: 10 min
Cooking time: 20 min

Nutrition:
Calories: 120
Points: 3
F: 6g, P: 15g, C: 3g.

Ingredients:
- 10oz fresh crab, chopped
- 2 cups fish stock
- 1 cup cubed carrots
- 2 shallots, diced
- 2 garlic cloves, minced
- 1 tbsp thyme
- 1 tbsp sage
- salt and pepper

Recipe:
1. Mix all the ingredients in your Instant Pot.
2. Seal and cook on Stew for 20 minutes.

PARSNIP AND GINGER SOUP

Serves: 6
Prep time: 10 min
Cooking time: 20 min

Nutrition:
Calories: 80
Points: 1
F: 6g, P: 2g, C: 11g.

Ingredients:
- 4lbs parsnip, peeled and diced
- 4 cups vegetable stock
- 1 large onion, diced
- 2 cloves garlic, minced
- 3tbsp minced ginger
- 2tbsp olive oil
- salt and pepper

Recipe:
1. Warm the oil in the base of your Instant Pot.
2. Soften the onion for 5 minutes.
3. Brown the parsnip in the olive oil and onion.
4. Add all the other ingredients.
5. Put the lid on and cook at high pressure for 20 minutes.
6. Blend.

Dessert

CHOCOLATE LOAF

Serves: 8
Prep time: 10 min
Cooking time: 10 min
Nutrition:
Calories: 300
Points: 7
F: 12g, P: 6g, C: 45g.
Ingredients:
- 1¾ cups unbleached all-purpose flour
- 1 cup condensed milk
- 1 cup water
- ½ cup brown sugar
- ½ cup chocolate chips
- ¼ cup honey
- 2 tablespoons vegetable oil
- 2 teaspoons baking powder
- 1 teaspoon pure vanilla extract
- ½ teaspoon ground cinnamon
- ¼ teaspoon ground nutmeg
- ¼ teaspoon ground allspice
- salt

Recipe:
1. Lightly oil a baking dish that will fit in the steamer basket of your Instant Pot.
2. In a bowl, mix the flour, baking soda, baking powder, salt and spices.
3. In another bowl combine the milk, honey, sugar, vanilla, and oil.
4. Fold the wet mixture into the dry mixture until smooth.
5. Fold in the chocolate chips.
6. Pour the batter into the baking tray and put the tray in your steamer basket.
7. Pour the water into the base of your Instant Pot and lower the steamer basket.
8. Seal and cook on Steam for 10 minutes.

COFFEE FLOAT

Serves: 6
Prep time: 5 min
Cooking time: 10 min

Nutrition:
Calories: 250
Points: 7
F: 20g, P: 7g, C: 32g.

Ingredients:
- 1 pint double chocolate ice cream
- 1 pint chocolate chip ice cream
- 4 cups hot brewed coffee

Recipe:
1. Combine coffee and chocolate ice cream in your Instant Pot.
2. Seal and cook on Stew 10 minutes.
3. Release the pressure quickly, pour into mugs. Top with a scoop of chocolate chip ice cream.

CHILI CHOCOLATE

Serves: 4
Prep time: 5 min
Cooking time: 10 min

Nutrition:
Calories: 200
Points: 6
F: 15g, P: 5g, C: 12g.

Ingredients:
- 4 cups milk
- ½ cup dark chocolate chips
- ¼ cup brown sugar
- 1tbsp cinnamon
- Pinch of cayenne pepper

Recipe:
1. Mix all the ingredients in your Instant Pot.
2. Seal and cook on Stew 10 minutes.

CHAI FLOAT

Serves: 6
Prep time: 5 min
Cooking time: 10 min

Nutrition:
Calories: 250
Points: 7
F: 20g, P: 7g, C: 32g.

Ingredients:
- 1 pint cinnamon roll ice cream
- 1 pint plain vanilla ice cream
- 4 cups hot spiced chai

Recipe:
1. Combine chai and cinnamon ice cream in your Instant Pot.
2. Seal and cook on Stew 10 minutes.
3. Release the pressure quickly, pour into mugs. Top with a scoop of vanilla ice cream.

WHITE CHOCOLATE

Serves: 4
Prep time: 5 min
Cooking time: 10 min

Nutrition:
Calories: 200
Points: 6
F: 15g, P: 5g, C: 12g.

Ingredients:
- 4 cups milk
- ½ cup white chocolate chips
- ¼ cup honey
- 1tsp nutmeg
- 1tsp vanilla extract
- 1tsp cinnamon

Recipe:
1. Mix all the ingredients in your Instant Pot.
2. Seal and cook on Stew 10 minutes.

GRANOLA STUFFED APPLES

Serves: 6
Prep time: 5 min
Cooking time: 20 min

Nutrition:
Calories: 150
Points: 3
F: 4g, P: 2g, C: 32g.

Ingredients:
- 6 Granny Smiths, peeled and cored
- 1.5 cups granola
- ½ a cup apple juice
- Juice of 1 lemon
- 2 tablespoons light brown sugar or granulated natural sugar
- 1.5 tablespoons butter, cut into 6
- ½ teaspoon ground cinnamon

Recipe:
1. Stand your apples up in your Instant Pot. You may need to do two batches.
2. In a bowl combine the sugar, granola, and cinnamon.
3. Stuff each apple with the granola and top with butter.
4. Pour the apple juice around the apples.
5. Seal the Instant Pot and cook on Stew for 20 minutes.
6. Depressurize naturally.

BANANA BREAD

Serves: 4
Prep time: 10 min
Cooking time: 30 min

Nutrition:
Calories: 200
Points: 5
F: 11g, P: 5g, C: 60g.

Ingredients:
- 3 mashed overripe bananas
- 2 cups flour
- 1.5 cups sugar
- 1 cup water
- ½ cup melted butter
- 2 eggs, beaten
- 2tsp baking powder
- 1tbsp mixed spices

Recipe:
1. In a bowl, whisk together the butter, eggs, and sugar. Slowly add the spices and baking powder.
2. With a fork, add the bananas and flour.
3. Grease a tray that fits in your Instant Pot steamer basket.
4. Pour the dough into the tray.
5. Pour the water into your Instant Pot and lower the basket.
6. Put the tray inside.
7. Seal and cook on Steam 30 minutes.

CHEESECAKE PORRIDGE

Serves: 4
Prep time: 4 min
Cooking time: 13 min

Nutrition:
Calories: 130
Points: 3
F: 6g, P: 4g, C: 23g.

Ingredients:
- 3.5 cups skim milk
- 1 cup porridge oats
- ½ cup raisins
- ¼ cup demarera sugar
- 2oz cream cheese
- 2tbsp white sugar
- 1tbsp butter
- 1tsp cinnamon

Recipe:
1. Melt the butter in your Instant Pot.
2. Add the oats and toast 3 minutes.
3. Add the salt and milk.
4. Seal and cook for 10 minutes on Rice.
5. Depressurize naturally.
6. Add the raisins and mix well.
7. In a bowl, whisk together sugars, cinnamon, and cream cheese.
8. Stir into porridge.

POACHED PEARS AND GINGER

Serves: 6
Prep time: 15 min
Cooking time: 15 min

Nutrition:
Calories: 120
Points: 2
F: 0g, P: 3g, C: 27g.

Ingredients:
- 2.5 cups apple juice
- 6 pears, peeled
- ¼ cup brown sugar
- ¼ cup crystallized ginger
- 1 cinnamon stick
- 2tsp grated ginger
- salt

Recipe:
1. Warm the juice, ginger, sugar, and salt in the Instant Pot.
2. Add the remaining ingredients.
3. Seal and cook on Stew for 15 minutes.
4. Depressurize naturally.
5. Remove the pears.
6. Warm the sauce to thicken it as desired.

APRICOT TAPIOCA PUDDING

Serves: 4
Prep time: 5 min
Cooking time: 13 min

Nutrition:
Calories: 230
Points: 6
F: 6g, P: 3g, C: 45g.

Ingredients:
- 2.5 cups milk
- ½ cup diced apricots
- ½ cup tapioca pearls, dry
- ½ cup brown sugar
- ¼ cup apricot jam

Recipe:
1. Mix all the ingredients in your Instant Pot.
2. Seal and cook on Stew for 13 minutes.
3. Depressurize naturally.

SPICED APPLESAUCE

Serves: 6
Prep time: 5 min
Cooking time: 25 min

Nutrition:
Calories: 230
Points: 4
F: 0g, P: 1g, C: 55g.

Ingredients:
- 2½ pounds apples, peeled, cored, diced
- ½ cup apple cider
- ⅓ cup brown sugar
- 1 teaspoon ground cinnamon
- Pinch of salt

Recipe:
1. Mix all the ingredients in your Instant Pot.
2. Seal and cook on Stew for 25 minutes.
3. Depressurize naturally.
4. Mash.

STEWED APPLES

Serves: 6
Prep time: 5 min
Cooking time: 10 min

Nutrition:
Calories: 200
Points: 3
F: 0g, P: 2g, C: 35g.

Ingredients:
- 6 chopped cooking apples
- 1 cup apple juice
- ½ cup brown sugar
- ½ cup raisins
- 2tbsp cinnamon

Recipe:
1. Put the apples in the base of your Instant Pot.
2. In a jug, combine the juice, sugar, raisins, and cinnamon.
3. Pour over the apples.
4. Seal and cook on Stew 10 minutes.

TAPIOCA PINA COLADA

Serves: 6
Prep time: 5 min
Cooking time: 10 min

Nutrition:
Calories: 200
Points: 4
F: 2g, P: 3g, C: 32g.

Ingredients:
- ½ cup dry tapioca pearls
- 1.5 cups coconut milk
- ½ cup pineapple juice
- ½ cup sugar

Recipe:
1. Mix all the ingredients in your Instant Pot.
2. Seal and cook on Rice 10 minutes.

CHOCOLATE CHEESECAKE

Serves: 6
Prep time: 15 min
Cooking time: 30 min

Nutrition:
Calories: 350
Points: 9
F: 16g, P: 13g, C: 38g.

Ingredients:
- 1 cup heavy cream
- 16oz cream cheese
- 1/2 cup chocolate cookie crumbs
- 1/2 cup sugar
- 2 whisked eggs
- 1oz dark chocolate
- 1tbsp butter
- 1tbsp cocoa powder
- 1tbsp vanilla mix

Recipe:
1. Mix the cookie and cinnamon and pack into the base of a greased heatproof pan that fits your steamer basket.
2. Melt chocolate and butter together.
3. Whisk together the cream cheese, cream, chocolate mix, sugar, and eggs. Add cocoa and vanilla slowly.
4. Pour the cheese mix over the crumbs.
5. Put the tray on the steaming basket and lower into your Instant Pot.
6. Cook on Steam 30 minutes.

APPLE CRUMB CAKE

Serves: 8
Prep time: 5 min
Cooking time: 20 min

Nutrition:
Calories: 200
Points: 5
F: 12g, P: 15g, C: 25g.

Ingredients:
- 2 cups applesauce
- 2 cups panko breadcrumbs
- 1 cup butter
- 1 cup water
- 3oz sugar
- 2tsp cinnamon
- 1tsp nutmeg
- 1/4tsp salt

Recipe:
1. Mix the dough with all but the water, and pour it into a greased or lined baking tray that fits in your steamer basket.
2. Add the water to your Instant Pot.
3. Put the dish in the steamer basket, insert the basket into the Instant Pot, and seal.
4. Cook on Steam for 20 minutes.

Conclusion

Over the course of this book we have seen how to combine the Weight Watchers program with Instant Pot cooking to make healthy eating a breeze. I hope that with these resources, yoyo dieting becomes a thing of the past for you, and you can finally enjoy life to the fullest whilst eating a healthy, wholesome, mostly home-cooked diet.